Medical Terminology

Learn to Pronounce, Understand, and Memorize Over 2000 Medical Terms

Notice

The information in this guide has been deemed to be as accurate as possible. Information on conditions, terms, and other concepts may change based on standards in the medical community.

Table of Contents

Introduction

Thank you for purchasing this book on medical terminology. The medical terms that you will encounter in a hospital or any other medical treatment center can be complicated and often hard to remember. It is not difficult for nurses, doctors and other health professionals to learn them gradually. While in the work environment, you will encounter terms ranging from specific procedures to the names of diseases. You will need to know these terms to complete different tasks in a medical environment.

Individual chapters in this book are dedicated to various parts of the body. The medical terms focus on body systems, such as the cardiovascular, digestive, endocrine, lymphatic, nervous, and skeletal systems. Each chapter includes information on the different prefixes, suffixes, and root words, which are used to identify medical terms. Each term that is difficult to pronounce has a pronunciation beside it. Proper pronunciations are necessary to appear knowledgeable while working in the medical field.

Other chapters include abbreviations that may be utilized in a report, such as symbols that make it easier for data to be conveyed in a table format. Various additional tips are included in this guide to help you remember these terms. You will notice that this book is very thorough and detailed and you will come across more than two thousand terms in this guide. You can also use this information to help you with any exams or tests that you plan on completing in the future.

An Index is included at the end of the paperback version of this book but not in the ebook version due to size limits.

Chapter 1 – Cardiovascular System

The cardiovascular system refers to the heart and the blood vessels. The terms in this chapter relate to the process by which blood is pumped and moved throughout the body. This includes the function of veins and blood vessels in the body. All segments in the cardiovascular system will redirect towards the heart based on the functionality of organs.

Some tests and readouts are included and may be used by medical staff. These tests relate to how the body functions and what readouts would be produced in a test that is ideal and normal. The test numbers help identify what treatments need to be carried out to facilitate a person's health.

aa. (eh-eh-)

An abbreviation for the arteries.

AAA

Abdominal aortic aneurism. This is an enlargement of the aorta, the blood vessel needed for delivering blood. The enlargement appears around the level of the abdomen.

Abdominal aorta (eh-or-tah)

The section of the aorta that descends through the diaphragm and into the abdomen.

ABI

Ankle-brachial index. This is the ratio of the blood pressure in the ankle to the blood pressure in the brachium or upper arm. Lower blood pressure in the ankle suggests the arteries are blocked or partially blocked due to peripheral artery disease.

ABO

The general classification of blood types. Blood may be identified as A, B, AB, or O. The blood group is based on the presence or absence of the A and B antigens. Type O appears when both of these antigens are absent. Type AB appears when both of those antigens appear. The type of blood determines the ability of the blood to process particular glycoproteins in the red cells.

aBP (eh-bee-pee)

Arterial blood pressure. The pressure is measured by a cuff that tightens around the upper arm. The pressure may be analyzed with the systolic and diastolic numbers reflecting how the heart functions.

AC

An anticoagulant.

Acanthocytes (eh-can-tho-cites)

Erythrocytes that have spiny projections on their bodies. These produce a thorny look.

Accelerated Idioventricular Rhythm

An automatic ectopic ventricular rhythm that produces a ventricular rate of about 50 to 100 beats per minute. The rhythm may be triggered for a few seconds, although it might last for up to a minute.

ACE

Angiotensin-converting enzyme. The enzyme controls the volume of fluids throughout the body, thus controlling blood pressure levels.

ACE Inhibitor

A drug that will lower blood pressure levels by inhibiting ACE production. The process allows blood flow to increase. The drug may help control hypertension or congestive heart failure.

Acebutolol (ace-bu-toe-lol)

A beta-blocker drug that treats hypertension. This may also assist in treating angina pectoris or irregular rhythm. The drug helps to improve how blood flows to the heart.

ACLS

Advanced cardiac life support. This is the treatment for a patient following a significant cardiovascular episode.

Adams-Stokes Syndrome

A condition caused by the heart being partially blocked. Fainting will occur regularly due to the condition.

Adenoid (eh-den-oid)

An enlarged portion of lymphatic tissue found behind the back of the nose or throat. The mass may impair speaking and other actions, although it may also trigger some heart-related issues.

Advanced Cardiac Life Support (ACLS)

A form of support that requires advanced treatments to help control significant cardiovascular episodes, including cardiovascular arrest. The process entails the urgent treatment of significant physical concerns brought upon by struggles of the heart. The process is used particularly for those who have become unconscious due to the cardiovascular issue in question.

AED

Automated external defibrillator. The device will produce an electric shock to the heart through the chest. The unit may be portable but will require precise control to ensure the device is used properly. People who have been trained in CPR or medical professionals may use an AED.

Afib/AF (eh-fib)

Atrial fibrillation. The condition is noted by an irregular heart rate. The rate may be elevated and causes poor blood flow. The heart will experience uncontrolled electric signals, thus triggering difficulties in its operation.

Afibrogenemia (eh-fib-ro-gen-ee-mee-ah)

A condition noted by a lack of fibrinogen in the blood. The blood will not clot due to the lack of the fibrinogen protein. The condition is rare and genetic in nature.

AHF

Antihemophilic factor. The compound is a protein responsible for blood clotting.

AIHA

Autoimmune hemolytic anemia. Red blood cells are destroyed faster than they are produced.

AIVR

Accelerated idioventricular rhythm, a ventricular rhythm from 40 to 120 beats per minute. The condition affects the cardiac ventricle.

Alprostadil (al-pro-sta-dill)

A vasodilator agent. The drug increases peripheral blood flow. The drug is used mainly for the treatment of impotence, but it may also help control cardiovascular issues.

AMI

Acute myocardial infarction also called a heart attack. Blood flow is blocked at the heart muscle, thus causing pains and tightness in the chest. The condition may impact the coronary artery.

Anacrotism (ah-nah-cro-tizm)

A secondary notch that develops in the pulse curve. A pulse tracing may be conducted to identify the issue.

Anaerobic (an-ah-er-oh-bick)

Activity in the heart that occurs without oxygen.

Anemia (ah-nee-mee-ah)

A condition where the blood does not include enough hemoglobin or erythrocytes, or red blood cells. This may be noticed as some of the blood cells will appear misshapen.

Aneurysm (an-ur-ism)

A condition where a blood vessel wall dilates. The aneurysm may include a sac-like appearance. The spot is weak and is at risk of rupturing.

Angina Pectoris (an-gi-nah pec-taur-is)

Chest pains that develop in the heart muscle. This is due mostly to ischemia or a lack of blood being supplied to the muscle.

Angiocardiography (an-gee-oh-car-dee-awgra-fee)

A radiographic test on the heart and vessels in the area. A contrast dye must be injected in the area to allow the test to be completed.

Angiography (an-gee-awg-ra-fee)

A procedure where a blood vessel is repaired. In this case, the vessel is widened after it has become narrow. A catheter is used in the process.

Angioscope (an-gee-oh-scope)

An endoscope that enters the body to review the insides of blood vessels.

Angiostenosis (an-gee-oh-sten-oh-sis)

A condition where a blood vessel narrows.

Angiotensin (an-gee-oh-ten-sin)

A series of peptides in the blood that cause hypertension and the constriction of veins.

Ankle Brachial Index

A measure of the ratio between the systolic blood pressure in an ankle and the same measure in an arm. The higher of the two blood pressures in the ankles is divided by the higher of the pressures of the arm pressures. The measure helps identify if cardiovascular disease is forming around the peripheral parts of the body.

Anticoagulants (an-ty-co-ag-uh-lints)

Drugs that prevent blood clotting, specifically by stopping the coagulation of the blood. By using an anticoagulant, the body's clotting time will decrease. This may assist in allowing blood to flow properly and reduces the risk of extensive clots forming in various parts around the body.

Antifibrinolytic (an-ty-fib-rin-oh-li-tic)

An agent that prevents a blood clot from breaking down.

Antihypertensive

A drug that reduces blood pressure levels to alleviate hypertension.

Aorta

A series of arteries that start at the left ventricle of the heart.

Aortic Aneurysm

A dilation found in the aortic wall. This may have a sac or balloon-like appearance.

Aortic Coarctation

A congenital heart issue where the aorta becomes narrow. The issue prevents the body from being able to handle blood flow correctly.

Aortic Stenosis (sten-oh-sis)

A condition where the aortic valve opening becomes narrow. Blood is unable to flow from the left ventricle to the aorta as usual.

Aortic Valve

A valve between the aorta and left ventricle. The valve prevents blood from flowing back into the left ventricle.

Aortic Valve Regurgitation

A condition where the aortic valve fails and blood flows into the left ventricle from the aorta. This may include the heart receiving blood that has been impacted by an inappropriate amount of oxygen that may impede the production of the heart's regular functions.

APA

Antipernicious anemia factor. Cobalamin or vitamin B12 is the most common factor that may help treat pernicious anemia.

Aplastic Anemia (eh-plas-tik)

A form of anemia where the bone marrow cannot produce enough blood elements.

Arrhythmia (ar-ith-me-ah)

A condition where the heart's beating rhythm becomes abnormal.

Arterial Blood Gas

A gas that will test oxygen, carbon dioxide, and pH levels in the blood.

Artery

A blood vessel that carries blood from the heart.

Arterioles

Smaller arteries found between the muscular arteries and the capillaries.

Arteriolosclerosis

A condition where the walls of the arteries become thick.

Arteriosclerosis

An occurrence of the arterial walls becoming thick and may become stiff.

Arteriostenosis

An event where the artery walls become narrow. The condition will immediately reduce how well blood flows and may potentially lead to some failures in the body depending on the intensity of the issue.

Arteritis

Inflammation in the arteries. The condition may cause the arteries to stop functioning as well as possible.

AS

Aortic stenosis. The aorta becomes narrow causing the heart to weaken while triggering fatigue.

ASD

Atrial septal defect. A birth defect that causes a hole to develop in the atria. The upper chambers of the heart are not controlled properly. An ASD may close on its own, but some larger ones require surgical treatment.

Asystole

A lack of cardiac functionality in the heart. This includes a lack of electrical functionality.

Atherectomy

A procedure where a catheter removes plaque from the arteries.

Atherosclerosis (ath-er-scl-er-oh-sis)

A condition where the arterial walls have lost their elasticity due to plaque developing in the area.

Atorvastatin

A drug that reduces cholesterol levels in the blood.

Atria

Upper chambers of the heart. These chambers receive blood flow from the body.

Atrial Flutter

An irregular heart rhythm. The heart may operate quickly and become a greater risk to the health of the heart.

Atrioventricular Node (ah-tree-oh-ven-trick-u-lur)

A series of muscle fibers around the bottom part of the right atrium. The muscles regulate the production of electrical signals to the ventricles. This prevents rapid functions in the atria while also ensuring that the atria empty properly.

Atrium

One of the two upper chambers in the heart. The left atrium links to the lungs and the right leads to the venous circulation area. The atria (the plural term) will receive blood and will pump that blood to the ventricles when the heart muscle contracts.

AUL

Acute undifferentiated leukemia. This is a form of blood cancer that originates in the bone marrow and may influence the production of blood cells and the workings of the cells.

Auscultation

The use of a stethoscope to hear sounds from the heart or other organs in the diagnostic process. The process involves an analysis of how well the heart is functioning and can give an indication of what may develop in the body.

Avascular (ah-vas-cue-lur)

A part of the body that is not receiving enough blood. This may be due to the blood vessels not working properly.

AVB

Atrioventricular block. The functionality between the atria and ventricles will be inhibited.

AVR

Accelerated ventricular rhythm. A ventricular rhythm that is faster than expected or faster than normal.

Bacteremia (back-ter-ee-mia)

A condition where bacteria can be found in the blood.

Bacterial Endocarditis

Inflammation within the lining of the heart or its valves.

Baroreceptor

A nerve ending in the heart that is sensitive to blood pressure changes.

Basophils (base-oh-fils)

A series of leukocytes that are common in an inflammatory response. These will develop a blue-black appearance when a contrast dye is introduced.

BBB

Bundle branch block. Electrical impulses on one part of the heart are not working properly. This may be due to a delay or a blockage.

BCLS

Basic cardiac life support. This is the first form of life support that is used on heart patients and may include CPR and AED support. First aid services may also be part of the support process.

Beta-Blocker

A drug that will slow the body's heart rate. By reducing the stress on the heart, blood pressure levels are likely to drop.

Blood Cell

A cell that is found in the blood.

Blood Clot

A mass that is formed in the body due to blood coagulation.

Blood Coagulation

A process where various blood factors interact with each other. The result is a blood clot.

Blood Plasma

The liquid part of blood. The fluid helps keep the blood cells whole and in suspension and includes moving proteins and cells throughout the entire body.

Blood Pressure

A measure of the pressure of blood around the arteries and veins. This may also influence the chambers of the heart.

Blood Vessels

Any kind of vessel responsible for transferring blood throughout the body.

Bone Marrow

A tissue that is found inside bone cavities. Bone marrow is necessary for producing all types of blood cells.

BPd

Diastolic blood pressure. The second number listed on a blood pressure test, the BPd is a measure of pressure in the blood vessels in between heartbeats.

BPs

Systolic blood pressure. The first number in a blood pressure test, the BPs is the pressure in the arteries as the heart muscle contracts.

Brachial Artery

An artery that branches off the axillary artery. This artery leads to the radial and ulnar arteries.

Bradycardia (bray-dee-car-de-ah)

An arrhythmia that occurs when the heart rate goes below 50 beats per minute. The condition is likely to occur among adults.

Bruit

A murmur that is heard when the carotid artery takes in more blood than expected.

Bundle Branch Block

A heart blockage where electrical signals to the ventricles are not moving properly.

Bundle of HIS

Cells that will cause electrical impulses to move from the atrioventricular node and then to the ventricles.

CABG

Coronary artery bypass graft. The process restores the blood flow to an artery that has experienced obstructions.

CADE

Coronary artery disease.

Calcium Channel Blocker

A drug that prevents calcium influx from developing in cellular membranes. The blockers will keep hypertension under control by relaxing the functionality of the heart.

Capillaries

Smaller blood vessels that transport nutrients and oxygen to the cells. The arterioles and venules are linked to the capillaries.

Capillary Fragility

A measure of how likely capillaries are to rupture or become damaged due to stress. This may be noticed by bleeding under the skin.

Catheterization

A process where a catheter is inserted into the heart tissue as a means of identifying conditions. This may also be utilized to control blocked arteries.

Cardiac Tamponade (tam-pon-ayd)

A compression developing in the heart due to fluid buildup.

Cardiomegaly (car-dee-oh-meg-allee)

Heart enlargement.

Cardiomyopathy

Disease of the heart muscle.

Cardiopulmonary Resuscitation

Also referred to as CPR, this is a procedure that entails manual heart massaging from outside the body and added mouth-to-mouth respirations. Professionals may be trained to conduct CPR.

Cardiotoxin

An outside compound that damages the heart.

Carditis

Inflammation in the heart.

Carotid Arteries (kar-aw-tid)

Arteries in the neck that move blood to the head. The arteries include internal and external branches.

Carotid Bruit

A murmur that may be felt on the carotid artery. This may suggest an increased risk of the person developing a stroke.

Carotid Stenosis

Narrowing of the carotid artery. This may be due to the development of plaque.

Cavogram

An angiogram of the vena cava.

CBC

Complete blood count. This is a measure of the approximate number of blood cells that appear in a sample, thus helping identify the general total of blood.

Celiac Artery

The artery that appears from the abdominal aorta. This leads to the left gastric artery and the splenic artery.

Central Line

An IV line that is inserted into a central vein in the body. The IV provides access to the bloodstream without interruption.

Centrifuge (sen-tri-fuge)

A material that will rotate an item in a fixed axis. The force produced separates materials in a space. It is used mainly for blood tests to identify concerns surrounding the development of certain bodies in the blood. The centrifuge will separate the materials in the blood to determine if a condition exists or the accuracy of a different test.

Cerebrovascular Disorder

A condition that causes blood to not flow to the brain.

CHB

Complete heart block. An unusual heart rhythm may develop due to the condition. There is no contraction moving through the atrioventricular node in the heart.

CHF

Congestive heart failure. The heart struggles to pump blood. This may be due to some blockages in the tissue.

Circle of Willis

A vascular network that appears around the base part of the brain. The network supplies blood to the region.

Clot

An insoluble mass that develops in a blood vessel that keeps blood from flowing properly. This may be formed by lymph or blood-related issues.

CoAg

Coarctation of the aorta.

Congenital Heart Defect

A heart condition that is present at birth.

Congestive Heart Failure

A condition where the heart is unable to pump blood properly.

Coronary Artery (core-aw-nair-ee)

The artery that moves blood from the aorta to the heart muscles.

Coronary Artery Disease

A condition where the blood flow through the coronary artery is reduced. Fat deposits form as plaques in the coronary artery. The deposits will progressively restrict blood flow, thus preventing blood from moving into the heart. The condition may result in a heart attack if not treated accordingly.

Coronary Occlusion

A lack of blood flow moving through a coronary artery.

Coronary Thrombosis

Clotting of blood in the coronary artery. This may result in heart failure.

Coumadin

A medication that prevents blood clots from developing. This may be prescribed for Afib. This can be found under the Jantoven name.

CVP

Central venous pressure. The blood pressure in the venae cavae around the right atrium. This is a measure of the ability of blood to return to the heart while the heart pumps blood back into the arteries.

DBP

Diastolic blood pressure. This is the second number on a blood pressure measurement. It is the pressure in the arteries as the heart is resting in between beats.

Defibrillation

A process where an electronic device helps produce an electric shock to the heart. This is to help restore the natural cardiac rhythm. The electric current may be delivered by a professional who has experience with handling a device, although proper training is required to ensure the treatment is done properly.

Diastole

The heart rhythm that develops as the ventricles are relaxed.

DIC

Disseminated intravascular coagulation. Blood clots develop inside blood vessels. The clotting factors are used up in certain areas, thus resulting in bleeding around other areas.

Dicrotic (die-crot-ick)

A heartbeat that develops with two peaks.

Digitalis (di-git-al-is)

A medicine that reduces the heart rate by improving heart contractions.

Diuretics (dye-ur-et-ix)

Medications that promote urination, thus reducing blood pressure. The medication keeps the fluid levels on blood vessels down. The urination will come from water in the cardiovascular system being slightly drained. The medication should only be consumed when prescribed by a doctor.

DVT

Deep vein thrombosis. This is a blood clot that appears in the leg or another deep vein.

Ebstein Anomaly

A congenital heart defect that can be noticed by the third and fourth heart sounds. The tricuspid valve will appear downward while the right atrium is enlarged.

ECG

Electrocardiogram. A process that helps identify the heart's muscular functioning. An ultrasound produces high-frequency sound waves to produce pictures of the heart tissue.

Ectopic Beats

Heartbeats that develop from electrical impulses. These may be produced outside of the SA note.

Ejection Click

A clicking sound that appears during auscultation. The condition may be a thickened aortic valve leaflet. The condition may also be something that happens when there is a blockage in one of the aortic valve leaflets.

EKG

Electrocardiogram. This is a measure of the electrical activity of the heart. This helps identify how well the heart is beating. This measures a P wave to identify proper atrial contractions and a T wave to see how the ventricles can relax. This may also be referred to as an ECG.

Elliptocytosis (el-lip-to-sign-toe-sis)

A condition where the body has more elliptical red cells in the blood than usual.

Embolectomy (em-bawl-eck-toe-mee)

An emergency procedure to remove a clot is removed from the body.

Embolism

A blockage in the blood vessel produced by a blood clot or other issue in the bloodstream.

Endarterectomy

A surgical procedure where the plaque in the lining of an artery is removed.

Endarteritis

Inflammation of the inside heart lining. The inflammation may also move into an artery that is very close to the heart. This may be caused by a bacterial infection.

Endocarditis (en-doh-car-die-tis)

Inflammation of the endocardium.

Endocardium

The inside layer of the heart. The membrane helps keep the chambers intact and will also produce the surface parts of the valves.

Endothelium (en-doh-the-le-um)

A layer of tissue that lines the heart, blood vessels, and other cavities in the body.

Eosinophil (ee-os-in-oh-fil)

A white blood cell responsible for fighting diseases.

Epicardium (ep-i-car-dium)

The inside layer of the pericardium, the tissue that covers the heart.

Erythroblast (er-e-thro-blast)

An immature red blood cell. This may be found in the bone marrow.

Erythrocyte (er-e-thro-cite)

A red blood cell. The cell includes the hemoglobin pigment and transports oxygen and carbon dioxide to the tissues in the body.

Erythroid (er-ith-roid)

A reddish tone in the blood cell.

Erythromelalgia (er-ith-roe-mel-al-jia)

A condition that develops when the arteries are not functioning or forming correctly. This may cause reddening around the extremities and intense pains.

Erythropoietin (er-ith-roe-poe-et-in)

A hormone produced by the kidneys responsible for producing red blood cells. The hormone is required to ensure the cells function properly.

Fibrillation

Twitching of the muscle fibers. This may be caused by unusual electrical impulses in the heart.

Fibrin (fib-rin)

A protein generated by blood clotting. The fibrin is insoluble and will be produced from fibrinogen while the blood clotting process takes place. The fibrin will produce a mesh that will impact the flow of blood.

Fibrinogen (fib-rin-o-gen)

A blood plasma protein that comes from the liver that helps to clot blood. The fibrinogen forms the fibrin.

Hematocrit (hee-mat-oh-crit)

A measure of red blood cells and their volume to the total amount of blood. The measure may be analyzed through centrifugation.

HDL

High-density lipoprotein. This is a protein that transports fat molecules throughout the body. A level over 60 mg/dL is ideal. A person with a level under 40 mg/dL may be at risk of some heart concerns, although the LDL level in the body may also be a factor that influences how well the body works.

Heart Arrest

When the heartbeat stops. This may be brought upon due to blockages in the arteries surrounding the heart and their inability to function properly.

Heart Block

A blockage of cardiac impulses.

Heart Failure

The inability of the heart to pump enough blood for the body's functionality.

Heart Murmur

A sound that develops from vibrations generated by blood flowing in the heart. The sound should be relative to the blood that flows through a heart valve, although the murmur will be more noticeable when there is a concern that develops in the valve.

Heart Septum

A structure in the thin atrium septum that appears between the atria. This may also be the thick septum that appears between the ventricles.

Heart Valve

A tissue that keeps blood from moving from the ventricles to the atria.

Hemangioma (he-mang-gee-oh-mah)

A birthmark that develops due to blood vessels being formed near the skin. This may also be called a strawberry mark. The mark will grow in one's infancy, but the appearance sometimes dissipates over time.

Hematocrit

The percentage of red blood cells by volume in a sample. The total is usually around 47% for men and 42% for women, although a 5% differential can be used in the measurement process.

Hemochromatosis (he-moe-crow-ma-toe-sis)

A condition where the body absorbs an excessive amount of iron, thus causing organ damage.

Hemoglobin (hee-moe-glow-bin)

Proteins that carry oxygen in red blood cells. The protein contributes to the red color of the blood. An iron atom is bound to a heme group in each hemoglobin molecule.

Hemorrhage (hem-or-rhage)

Bleeding in a vessel. This may be external or internal in nature. The condition can occur in various vessels, although the concern is most commonly associated with the head.

Hemostasis (he-moh-stay-sis)

A process where the body suddenly stops a hemorrhage. This may develop from vessel contraction or coagulation among other factors.

Heparin (hep-air-in)

An anticoagulant. This is an injection that will decrease the body's ability to clot. The compound is not a blood thinner, although it may be referred to in some journals as one.

Hydremia (high-drim-ee-a)

Excess water in the blood. The condition may keep blood cells from moving with one another accordingly, thus causing fatigue and an inability to move proteins throughout the body as well as necessary.

Hyperlipidemia (high-pur-lip-eh-de-mee-ah)

A condition where the blood has excess fats or lipids. The condition may be a genetic or acquired disorder that includes fats, cholesterol deposits, and triglycerides.

Hypernatremia (hi-pur-nat-reem-ee-a)

A condition where the blood has excess sodium. The serum sodium concentration goes over 145 mmol/L. The condition would entail a decline in the total body water or TBW total that is relative to the electrolyte content in the body.

Hyperphosphatemia (high-pur-fos-fate-em-ee-a)

When the blood has high phosphate totals. The condition may also entail low calcium levels in the body, which will then produce muscle spasms. Part of this includes changes in how the heart functions.

Hypertension

A condition noted by high blood pressure. The condition is typically identified as blood pressure over 130/80 and can be even more significant if the total is at over 180/120. The condition does not have any symptoms.

Hypertriglyceridemia (high-pur-tri-gliss-er-ide-eem-ee-a)

When the blood has high triglyceride levels. The fatty molecule in the body becomes prominent and may result in atherosclerosis, and eventually lead to a person having an elevated risk of cardiovascular disease. The condition is common among those who may be obese, those who do not engage in enough physical activity, or those who have Type II diabetes or metabolic syndrome.

Hypocalcemia (high-poe-cal-ceem-ee-a)

Low calcium in the blood. The condition will be measured by the amount of calcium found in the blood plasma. The lack of calcium leads to the inability of the body to conduct its electrical functions. The condition may trigger numbness, tingling in the extremities, and cramps.

Hypokalemia (high-poe-cal-eem-ee-a)

Low potassium in the blood. This may be controlled by the kidneys. Hypokalemia may be the kidneys causing excess amounts of potassium to travel through the body through urine or sweat. Vomiting and nausea may develop.

Hyponatremia (high-poe-na-treem-ee-ia)

A lack of sodium in the blood often caused by an excess total of body fluids. The total is measured in the serum that has less than 136 mEq/L of sodium. The condition involves the water levels in the body being excessive.

Hyperfusion (hi-po-per-fu-sin)

Lack of blood flow in an organ.

Hypotension

Low blood pressure. The condition may cause dizziness or intense fatigue. The problem may be triggered by the heart and brain not communicating with each other properly, thus hindering the proper blood pressure rating in the body. A condition under 90/60 may be interpreted as hypotension.

Hypovolemia (high-poe-vole-ee-mah)

Low volume of blood circulation. The blood plasma level is too low.

Iilac Artery (ill-ee-ack)

A large artery developing from the abdominal aorta. There are two of these arteries in the body. The arteries help to move blood to the pelvis and legs.

Infarction

A condition where tissues die due to a lack of oxygen. This may be due to a lack of oxygenated blood moving through the body or an inability of the body to function properly.

Intracranial Embolism

Blockage of a blood vessel in the skull. This may be due to materials in the bloodstream not dissolving properly.

Ischemia (is-keem-e-ah)

Hypoperfusion is when blood vessels are obstructed. The condition prevents oxygen from moving properly, thus making it harder for cells to metabolize to keep tissues functional. The issue may be due to blood vessels not functioning properly. This may also be a general effect of CAD or coronary artery disease.

Ischemic Heart Disease

Chest pains that occur due to the heart not receiving blood. The condition may be noticed in people who engage in excess physical activities.

Jugular Vein

A vein in the neck that moves blood from the brain to the heart. Each side of the neck has an internal and external vein.

JVD

Jugular venous distention. Pressure levels in the jugular vein increase, thus causing a bulging effect. The condition may be a sign of added pressure that might keep the body from functioning properly.

JVP

Jugular venous pulse. This is the pressure that is identified in the venous system based on how the internal jugular vein is operating.

LDL

Low-density lipoprotein. The protein helps move fat molecules throughout the bloodstream. An excess total may result in heart failure and other related conditions. An LDL of 130 to 159 mg/dL implies that a person is at an elevated risk of significant conditions. A total of over 160 mg/dL is high.

Leukemia (lou-key-mee-a)

Cancer of the blood. The bone marrow is unable to produce healthy white blood cells. The condition may cause a fever and swelling in the lymph glands, although not all people who experience leukemia will develop symptoms. A blood test is required to identify the condition and if it is spreading or if it exists.

Leukocyte (lou-koe-site)

A white blood cell. The cell is noted for not having any color. The cell helps fight infections and enhance the functionality of the body's immune system. An excess of white blood cells may indicate an infection within the body.

Lymphocyte

A white blood cell that assists in the body's general immune response to an infection.

MAP

Mean arterial pressure. This is the average blood pressure in a single cardiac cycle and is measured based on systolic and diastolic blood pressure totals. This is a test used to identify the perfusion of blood to vital organs and may be used in lieu of a test involving systolic blood pressure.

MCH

Mean corpuscular hemoglobin. This is the mass of the hemoglobin for each red blood cell. The total is the amount of hemoglobin in a volume of blood and is not related to the number of red blood cells in that same volume sample.

MCV

Mean corpuscular volume. This is the average volume of red blood cells. The MCV should be around 80 to 96 fL/red cells in an adult body.

Megaloblastic Anemia (mega-low-blast-ick)

A form of anemia where the red blood cell count is low due to the body having too many large red blood cells. This may be caused by a lack of folate or cobalamin.

Megaloblast (may-gah-low-blast)

A red blood cell precursor that is very large in size. This may be found in people who have pernicious anemia.

Microvessels

Smaller blood vessels that are only visible through a microscope.

Mitral Stenosis

A condition where the mitral valve narrows. This may develop due to rheumatic fever at any age. The condition does not generate symptoms unless it is severe.

Mitral Valve (mee-trul)

A valve that appears between the left atrium and ventricle.

Mitral Valve Prolapse

A condition where the mitral valve appears to protrude slightly. Blood may flow back into the heart due to the condition.

Mitral Valve Stenosis

When the mitral valve becomes narrow.

Monocyte

A leukocyte that assists white blood cells in removing old tissues and with clearing out cancer cells. This may also help control the body's immunity response. The cell is produced within the bone marrow.

MRA

Magnetic resonance angiography. The process helps identify how blood vessels operate and if they are visibly active. The arteries are reviewed through a visual scan to identify any unusual functions in the tissues and to identify the issues that the body might develop at this point. Not to be confused with an MRI, a similar scan that focuses on other parts of the body.

Myelodysplastic Syndrome

A cancer form where the blood cells that have not formed properly. The blood cells in the bone marrow are not functioning properly.

Myocardial Infarction (my-oh-card-e-ul)

The death of heart tissue due to a lack of blood. This may also be called a heart attack.

Myocardial Ischemia

A condition where the cardiac function stops due to blood flow not moving to the muscle tissue in the heart.

Myocarditis

Inflammation of the heart muscle, usually due to an infection. The condition will influence the middle part of the heart wall and can lead to shortness of breath and chest pain. Some patients may also experience an irregular heartbeat.

Myocardium (my-oh-car-de-um)

The heart muscle. The muscle produces contractions needed to pump blood from the heart to the lungs and other critical organs. The system is connected to the circulatory system.

Neovascularization (knee-oh-vas-cue-lur-eh-zay-shun)

The body's natural production of blood cells. The process is the development of new microvascular networks to help produce red blood cells.

Neutropenia (new-troe-pee-nee-ah)

A decline in the number of neutrophils needed to allow blood to flow. The condition may develop due to some cancer treatments.

Neutrophils (new-troh-filz)

White blood cells respond to infections.

Nitroglycerin (nigh-tro-glis-er-in)

A medication that may help dilate veins and control angina pectoris.

Normotensive

A condition where the patient has a normal blood pressure rate.

Occlusion

When a blood vessel is blocked.

P Wave

A wave noticed in a heart readout. The wave will note atrial depolarization.

PAC

Premature atrial contraction. This may be noted in a test based on when heartbeats occur at incorrect times.

Pacemaker

A device that may be implanted in a patient's body. The device produces electric impulses to trigger regular heart functionality.

PAD

Peripheral arterial disease. The blood vessels constrict, thus keeping blood from flowing to the limbs as normal.

PAF

Platelet-activating factor. The compound will trigger the production of platelets needed to help produce healthy functions in the body.

Palpation

A process where the fingers are used on the patient's chest during an exam. A light amount of pressure may be applied. The sensation felt by the patient within his/her body may be intense.

Paroxysmal Atrial Tachycardia (pear-ox-is-mal)

An irregular heartbeat that causes the heart rate to increase.

Paroxysmal Supraventricular Tachycardia

A rapid heartbeat may occur suddenly without prediction. The heartbeat may last for a few seconds, but it could also go on for hours depending on how the patient responds.

Patent Ductus Arteriosus

An extra blood vessel that appears after birth. This is an opening that develops between the blood vessels that normally lead from the heart. The condition may be small and could shrink over time. It may stay open for a little longer and cause excess blood to flow to the lungs, thus potentially requiring surgery.

Perfusion

The process where blood is delivered to the capillaries.

Pericardial Effusion

The development of fluid within the pericardium. This may be due to an elevated amount of sodium causing the fluid to increase in volume.

Pericardial Fluid

Watery fluid develops in the serous and visceral pericardium around the heart.

Pericardial Friction Rub

An added sound that may be the heart in pericarditis. The condition produces a squeaking sound.

Pericardiocentesis (pear-e-car-dee-oh-cen-tee-sis)

A puncture in the pericardium that causes fluid to leak from the area.

Pericarditis (pear-eh-car-dye-tis)

Inflammation of the pericardium. The condition prevents the heart from being able to stay in its regular place. Swelling may develop in the area. Irritation may also be a concern.

Pericardium (pear-i-car-dee-um)

The thin sac that covers the heart. Fluid develops between the layers to help lubricate the tissue, thus allowing for regular functionality.

Periphlebitis (pear-e-fleh-bie-tiss)

Inflammation of tissues surrounding a vein.

Pernicious Anemia

Anemia caused by a lack of cobalamin or vitamin B12, also known as Addison's anemia. The body is unable to absorb the cobalamin, thus causing a decline in the number of red blood cells in the body. The issue may trigger fatigue in some patients.

Phlebography

A review of veins in the body, particularly in the legs. A catheter allows for a contrast agent to be injected through a catheter. The test is used to identify deep vein thrombosis.

Phlebotomy

A process used for drawing blood from the vein for testing purposes. Venipuncture will be produced with finger pricks to collect small quantities of blood.

Phonocardiogram

A review of the heart sound amplitude. The test reviews a few heartbeats to see how the tissue is functioning. The test includes a full cardiac cycle and can record any murmurs that develop.

Plaque (plak)

A fatty development on an arterial wall. The plaque may develop over time and build up to where the artery will not be capable of moving blood properly, thus leading to cardiac arrest.

Plasma

The liquid part of the blood. The compound includes nutrients, particularly glucose. This also assists in blood clotting.

Platelet (plat-lit)

A part of the blood that will clot to keep blood vessels from leaking. The compounds are used mainly for handling injuries.

Pleocytosis (puh-lee-oh-sigh-toe-sis)

A high number of cells found in cerebrospinal fluid.

Polymorphonuclear (pol-e-mor-pho-new-clear)

A condition where the number of white blood cells in the body is abnormally high.

PNH

Paroxysmal nocturnal hemoglobinuria. The immune system will start destroying healthy red blood cells. The condition will cause fatigue and may be difficult to treat with some drugs.

Polycythemia (pol-e-ceh-the-mee-a)

A rise in the number of red blood cells in the body. This may be measured based on the hematocrit or volume of red blood cells in the body. An elevated total may be a sign of a blood clot or an elevated risk of a heart attack or stroke.

Profunda

Blood vessels that are inside the body tissues that need to be served.

PSVT

Paroxysmal supraventricular tachycardia. The heart rate becomes faster around the two lower chambers of the heart. The electrical impulses of the heart are disrupted due to the condition. This may result in some heart palpitations, although not all patients are likely to experience symptoms due to the condition.

PTCA

Percutaneous transluminal coronary angioplasty. This is a procedure needed to open a blocked coronary artery, thus allowing blood to circulate properly into the heart muscle. The treatment is minimally invasive.

PTT

Partial thromboplastin time. The blood test assists in identifying how long it would take for the blood to clot as a test chemical is applied to a blood sample. The PTT is measured in seconds and should be from 25 to 35 seconds. This means that the clotting should happen within that time period. A high number of seconds suggests that it is taking longer for the body to produce clots and could indicate that the body could be at a high risk of excess clots and a lack of blood flow to the proper tissues.

Pulmonary Artery (pull-mun-arie)

An artery that moves blood from the right ventricle to the lungs.

Pulmonary Circulation

The movement of blood in the lungs.

Pulmonary Valve

A valve that appears where the right ventricle meets with the pulmonary artery.

Pulmonary Valve Regurgitation

The flow of blood back from the pulmonary artery to the right ventricular artery. This may be due to the pulmonary valve leaking.

Pulmonary Valve Stenosis

A narrowing of the pulmonary valve. Blood will not flow from the right ventricle into the pulmonary artery at the same rate as earlier.

Pulmonary Vein

A vein that moves oxygenated blood from the lungs back to the heart's left atrium.

Pulse

An analysis of how well blood is pumping. The pulse is a measure of how an artery can expand and contract. The process occurs as blood pumps from the heart. The pulse is measured in the number of beats per minute that are reviewed in the test. A normal resting rate is 60 to 100 beats per minute for most other people and could be around 40 beats more per minute for athletes. A high resting rate may be dangerous.

Purkinje Fiber (purr-kin-jay)

A muscle fiber in the heart that assists in producing the cardiac impulses from the atrioventricular node to the ventricles, thus allowing the muscle to contract.

PVC

Premature ventricular contraction. This is an added heartbeat that appears in the ventricles. The beat will disrupt the natural ability of the heart to pump blood properly.

Pylethrombosis (pie-lee-throm-boe-sis)

Thrombosis developing in the portal vein or the associated branches. The condition is caused by an infection.

QRS Complex

A review of an EKG that identifies ventricular functionality and cases where the vein is not functioning as effectively as usual. The measurement is for the main spike that may be found on an EKG line.

Radial Artery

An artery that starts in the forearm and ends around the brachial artery. The vein moves along other parts of the arm.

Raynaud's Disease

A condition where the body may feel numb in some cases. This is due to smaller arteries that transfer blood to the skin contracting quickly. The area may appear dark due to a lack of blood flow, and then red as the blood returns to the area.

RBC

Red blood cell count. The count is the number of cells in a sample of blood. An average RBC readout is 14 to 17 gm/dL for men or 12 to 15 gm/dL for women. A low total states that you do not have enough iron in the blood, thus keeping your body from producing enough red blood cells.

Reperfusion

The restoration of blood to ischemic tissue.

Restenosis

When stenosis occurs in an artery following proper treatment.

Reticulocyte (wre-tick-you-lo-site)

A new red blood cell that has not yet developed a nucleus. The cell may feature a granular look to its body.

Rhesus Factor

A protein on the surface of a red blood system. The protein may be identified in a blood test. In most cases, a person will have the Rhesus or Rh factor protein in their bloodstream. A person who does not have the Rh factor is Rh-negative.

Rheumatic Heart Disease

A condition that is caused following rheumatic fever. The heart may develop inflammation following the basic symptoms of the fever. The condition may develop following an improperly treated case of scarlet fever or strep throat.

S-T Segment

A segment that appears on an EKG that identifies the timing between ventricular depolarization and repolarization.

S1-4

The heart sounds that may be heard in a test. These range from the first to fourth sounds.

Semilunar Valve

The pulmonary or aortic valve. A series of cusps may be noticed in these parts.

Sepsis

A condition that develops when the immune system produces an excess reaction to an infection. The condition causes inflammation to develop throughout the body. Bacteria enter the bloodstream in this condition, thus impairing the body's ability to clear the toxins. Multiple organs may be damaged in this condition, and this may also lead to death.

Septal Defect

A hole found in the septum. The condition is congenital. This may heal on its own after birth, although this may also require surgical treatment if the condition appears well after birth.

Septicemia

An infection in the blood, or bacteremia. This is a technical name for sepsis.

Septic Shock

Sepsis that develops alongside hypotension. The condition may develop in spite of added fluids in the body.

Sinoatrial Node (sin-oh-eh-tree-al)

A mass of muscle fibers found in the right atrium. The contraction impulses are produced at the node and will move along the atrium. This is also called the SA node.

Serum

The blood plasma that appears after clotting proteins are removed. The serum is separated outward as blood coagulates.

Sick Sinus Syndrome

A concern suggesting that the sinus node is not functioning well enough to allow the natural pace-making functions of the heart. The condition is not a disease but is a sign that there may be a concern in the body that could influence how it functions and handles blood.

Sickle Cell Anemia

A form of anemia that is inherited. The red blood cells become rough in texture and will stick to one another. These cells will also develop sickle-like shapes. The cells will get stuck around the blood vessels, thus causing blockages around various parts of the body.

Sinoatrial Block

An electrical impulse that develops in the sinoatrial node. This occurs when the node is blocked before signals can get to the atrium.

Sinoatrial Node (sin-oh-ah-tree-al)

A series of muscle fibers found in the cardiac muscle. The fibers are in the upper right atrium.

Sinus Rhythm

A heart rhythm identified through an EKG reading. The total is a regular heartbeat based on the heart rate involved and the rhythm. The total should be from 60 to 100 beats per minute in most people, although this may be lower in a healthy athlete. A high total suggests there may be a concern in the body.

Souffle (sue-flay)

A blowing sound that may be heard through a stethoscope.

Spherocyte (s-feer-oh-site)

A small red blood cell with an excess amount of hemoglobin.

Spherocytosis (s-feer-oh-sigh-toe-sis)

A blood disorder identified by small red blood cells. The cells may include spherical shapes. The condition may produce fatigue and shortness of breath.

Splenic Artery (spleen-ick)

A large branch in the celiac trunk. The artery moves blood to the spleen, pancreas, and stomach.

Stasis (stay-sis)

A lack of blood or other important fluids in the body.

Stent

A small tube that expands arteries particularly narrowed ones.

Stress Test

A test that identifies how well the patient's blood pressure, heart rate, and other cardiovascular functions are operating. The test may use a treadmill or other device to see how well the patient responds to physical activity.

Stroke

A condition caused by a lack of blood functioning in the brain. The condition is noted by a lack of physical and neurological functionality. The condition may cause drooping in one part of the face and can cause a person to become unable to move normally. Appropriate treatment is required as soon as possible to prevent permanent brain damage from developing due to the issue.

Stroke Volume

A measure of blood pumped from a ventricle in one heartbeat. The ideal stoke volume is listed at 70 mL, although the best possible readout may vary based on the person who is being tested.

Sudden Cardiac Arrest

A sudden lack of cardiac activity. The condition is caused by a lack of electrical functionality and may be reversed if treated soon after the condition develops.

Supraventricular Tachycardia (sue-pra-ven-trick-u-lur tach-ee-car-de-ah)

When the heart rate is faster above the lower chambers. The electrical impulses in the heart will not function properly. Heart palpitations may develop in this case.

Syncope (sin-kope)

Fainting caused by a lack of blood in the brain. The condition causes a loss of consciousness.

Systole (sis-toll)

A point in heart contraction that occurs as blood moves from the systemic circulatory system into the lungs.

Systolic Blood Pressure

A measurement of the blood pressure as the heartbeats. This is the first number readout on a blood pressure test.

Systolic Murmur

A heart murmur that takes place during heart contraction. The sound appears between the first and second sounds.

Thrombocyte (throm-boh-cite)

Platelet. The tissue helps to prevent bleeding from developing.

Thrombocytopenia (throm-boh-cy-toe-pen-ee-ah)

A drop in the number of blood platelets in the blood. The test is a review of platelets in a blood sample. A total of fewer than 150,000 platelets per milliliter of blood is a sign of the condition. The condition increases the risk of the patient bleeding. The condition is too many platelets being destroyed at a time or the bone marrow not making enough platelets. The platelets may also be destroyed due to an enlarged spleen. Easy bruising may develop.

Thrombocytosis (throm-bo-seh-toe-sis)

An excess amount of platelets in the blood tissue. The condition may be primary where unusual bone marrow cells produce an excess of platelets, although the issue may also be secondary in nature. The issue will cause the patient's blood flow to decline due to an elevated number of clotting factors in the body. The condition develops when the body has more than 450,000 platelets in one milliliter of blood.

Thrombolysis (throm-bo-ly-sis)

A treatment process used to dissolve clots in blood vessels to prevent organs from being damaged. The treatment may require a surgical procedure to remove a vein clot. This can be done in the treatment of deep vein thrombosis.

Thrombolytic (throm-bo-ly-tic)

The process of breaking up a thrombus.

Thrombophilia (throm-bo-ph-e-lah)

A condition where the body is at an elevated risk of developing thrombosis.

Thrombosis (throm-boe-sis)

The development of a blood clot in a vessel. The condition keeps the circulatory system from developing the blood flow it requires. The condition may develop in the leg as deep vein thrombosis, although a more serious form of the clot may also form in the heart tissue.

Torsades De Pointes (taur-sod-es de pont)

A form of tachycardia that develops with a long QT interval. The EKG test readout will show that there is an irregularity in the regular heartbeat. The issue may trigger ventricular fibrillation in some patients. The condition will occur when the heart rate is between 200 and 250 beats per minute. The amplitude in the QRS complex may also change and twist over time.

Tourniquet (turn-i-ket)

A band that compresses a blood vessel. The band should be applied over a limb during the blood testing process to ensure the patient is at a reduced risk of experiencing bleeding from the injection site. The band may also go over a wound that is bleeding consistently.

Toxemia (tocks-em-e-ah)

Also known as blood poisoning. Bacteria develop in the blood. The condition reveals swelling or edema in the body, hypertension, and protein in the urine. The condition is more likely to develop in pregnant women.

Transfusion

A process where blood is transferred from one person to another.

Tricuspid Valve (try-cuss-pid)

A heart valve between the right atrium and ventricle. The valve will keep blood from flowing from the ventricle back into the atrium.

Tricuspid Valve Regurgitation

When the tricuspid valve fails to prevent blood from moving back to the right atrium from the right ventricle.

Tricuspid Valve Stenosis

When the opening to the tricuspid valve narrows. The condition is often produced by rheumatic fever.

Trigeminy (trig-em-in-e)

A condition where the EKG reveals three unique beat patterns. The condition may be two regular sinus beats alongside an unusual one at the end, or it may be the other way around.

VAD

Venous assist device. A tube that is inserted in a large vein. The tube may be used as a catheter to provide regular access to a vein without having to use a deep needle stick. This allows for the administration of proper nutrients and other important compounds to keep the body healthy.

Valsalva Maneuver (val-sal-vah)

A test where a person will attempt to exhale while one's airway is closed. This may involve closing the mouth and pinching the nose shut while attempting to press air out from the face. An otoscope is used in the ear to identify how the ear tissue changes during the effort. The process may help identify the changes in the body's heart rate and blood pressure during the process.

Varicose Vein (var-e-cose)

An enlarged vein that regularly appears in the leg. The vein has become snagged and is no longer straight. The tissue swells and is noticeable along the skin just under the surface. The condition is benign and the cause of the issue is unknown.

Vascular (vas-cu-lur)

Relating to a blood vessel.

Vasculitis (vas-cue-ly-tis)

Inflammation in a blood vessel.

Vasoconstriction (vas-oh-con-stric-shun)

When the blood vessel narrows from the muscular wall contracting in the vessels. The condition develops mainly in the arteries, although the arterioles may also be influenced.

Vasoconstrictor (vas-oh-con-stric-tur)

Drugs that will cause the blood vessels to constrict or narrow.

Vasodilation (vas-oh-die-lay-shun)

When the blood vessels widen.

Vasodilator (vas-oh-die-lay-tur)

A drug that dilates or expands the blood vessels. The opposite of a vasoconstrictor.

VCT

Venous clotting time. A measure of time it takes for the blood in a vein to clot. The blood in the vein is tested at 37 degrees Celsius and reviewed to identify how long it takes for the sample to clot. The average time for clotting should be from 8 to 15 minutes.

Vein (vain)

A vessel that carries blood from the capillary bed.

Venae Cavae (ven-ay cav-ay)

Two venous trunks that will transport blood to the heart. The interior venae cavae will take in blood from the lower body. The superior vanae cavae will move blood from the upper body.

Venous Insufficiency

When venous blood flow or return is impacted. The condition may occur in the legs, although it can develop in any place where the venous valves are not working properly.

Venous Thrombosis

The development of a blood clot in a vein.

Ventricles (ven-trick-uls)

Two heart chambers that take in blood from the atria. The ventricles will pump the blood to the circulatory systems.

Ventricular Fibrillation

Also called V-fib or VF - When excess and uncontrolled electrical impulses start to form in the ventricles. The condition may cause about 400 to 600 impulses per minute. This may be triggered by a heart attack and can cause low blood pressure and a reduced heart rate. The issue can keep cardiac functions from developing and may lead to death if not treated. An AED and CPR may be required to restore consciousness and heart functionality.

Ventricular Flutter

A condition where ventricular tachycardia develops quickly. This may include a large sine-wave that appears in the EKG readout. The total runs at 150 to 300 beats per minute. The condition may lead to ventricular fibrillation if not treated.

Ventricular Tachycardia

A fast heart rhythm that develops in the ventricles. The rhythm may be quick, but it will stay consistent. The issue develops mainly due to heart disease in older persons and may be elevated in those who regularly use over-the-counter decongestants. The condition may trigger fainting, dizziness, and shortness of breath. It is also known as VT.

VLDL

Very low-density lipoprotein. This type of lipoprotein contains more triglycerides than others. The compounds are needed to allow fats and cholesterol to move through the bloodstream. An excess may result in a significant threat to the body's natural rate of blood flow.

VSD

Ventricular septal defect. This is a hole that develops between the lower chambers. The condition will cause oxygen-rich blood to mix with oxygen-poor blood. The condition develops upon birth, although the wall should regularly close before the fetus is born. The defect may also close on its own, although a surgical procedure may be required depending on the situation.

vv

An abbreviation for the veins.

White Coat Hypertension

A condition where a person's blood pressure is elevated when it is taken in a clinic. It is unclear as to what causes the issue to develop.

WPW

Wolff-Parkinson-White syndrome. The condition develops when an added electrical pathway forms between the heart's chambers. The condition causes the heartbeat to be faster. The condition develops at birth and it may resolve itself over time. An electric shock may also be produced to restore the heart's rhythm if the condition is found in an adult.

Prefixes

Angio	Blood vessels
Ao	Aorta
Arteri	Artery
Arteriol	Smaller artery

Ather	Fatty deposits in the cardio system
Atri	Atrium
Bas	Basilar
Brady	Slow
Cardio	Heart
Coagul	Coaguation or clotting
Erythr	Red
Erythrocty	Red blood cell
Hemo	Blood
Hemat/o	Blood
Leuk/o	White
Myocardi	Myocardium
Pericardi	Pericardium
Phlebo	Vein
Plasmo	Plasma
Presby	Older age
Puls	Beating
Purpur	Purple in appearance
Rhe	The general flow or stream of the heart's functionality
Ser	Blood serum
Sphygmo	Pulse
Systol	Contraction
valv/o	vale
vas/o	vessel
vascul/o	blood vessel

ventricul/o   ventricle

Chapter 2 – Digestive System

The following chapter focuses on terms relating to digestive health. The digestive system refers to the structures, organs, and other parts of the body responsible for the breakdown of foods, the absorption of nutrients, and the body's ability to remove waste. The system is required to ensure the general health of the body and to restore its natural functions, although some disorders may develop that may cause some difficulties in how well the area may operate.

Some of the terms in this chapter refer to the compounds that a person may consume as a regular diet. These may influence how well the body responds to certain treatments and functions. These terms may relate to how well the body may develop, especially with deficits leading to some conditions.

Antibiotic-Associated Diarrhea (AAD)

Diarrhea that is triggered by the use of antibiotics. The condition may cause intense fatigue.

Abdominal Pain

Pains in the abdomen. This may be chronic in some patients and may cause uncomfortable feelings in other patients.

Abdominal Quadrant

A segment of the abdomen that is divided by a series of horizontal and vertical lines. These lines intersect at the umbilicus.

Abdominal Wall

The boundaries of the abdomen. This may include the skin, subcutaneous fat, muscles, and other areas of the body.

Abdominoplasty (ab-dom-in-oh-plas-tee)

A surgical procedure where excess fat and skin are removed from the abdomen. This is called a tummy tuck for how the process tightens the abdominal wall.

Acarbose (eh-car-bouse)

A drug that treats type 2 diabetes. The drug slows down the body's ability to digest complex carbohydrates.

Achlorhydria (eh-klor-high-drah)

A lack of hydrochloric acid in the emission of gasses.

Aerophagia (air-oh-fay-gee-ah)

When the person swallows more air than needed. This may be caused by anxiety or incorrect eating habits. The condition can cause an upset stomach and irritation in the body. This is also a repetitive condition.

Ageusia (agg-you-shah)

When a person loses the sense of taste. This may be due to the improper function of nerves that trigger sensations of taste.

Alimentary Canal (al-eh-men-tair-ee)

A passage point for food that goes from the mouth to the anus. The passage helps digest and absorb food.

Amino Acid

An organic compound that contains carboxyl and amine functioning groups. Amino acids may help build healthy body tissues.

Amylase (ah-mee-laise)

Enzymes that digest starches. The enzyme is found mainly in saliva and in the pancreatic fluid. The enzyme converts glycogen and starch into simple sugars.

Amylose (ah-meel-oze)

A soluble part of starch. This is a crystallized form of the compound that is soluble in water and makes up about a third of the starch that a person consumes.

Anal Canal (eh-null)

The end of the large intestine. This is where the intestine links up to the anus.

Anastomosis (ann-as-to-mos-sis)

A link that appears between two bodies. This is produced during a surgical procedure. In most cases, this may be a connection between the two halves of the intestines.

Anorexia Nervosa (an-or-ecks-ee-a nur-vo-sa)

An eating disorder that is a loss of appetite, thus causing the person to not eat anything. This may also be caused because a person is afraid of being overweight.

Antacid

A compound that controls acidity in the stomach. The drug neutralizes the production of acids in the stomach, although it may cause a pH imbalance if the body does not have enough acid.

Anthelmintic (an-thel-min-tick)

A compound that destroys a parasitic worm. This helps prevent the development of such worms.

Antidiarrheal (an-thai-die-ah-ree-al)

A drug that treats diarrhea. The drug may treat the symptoms of diarrhea, although the quality of the drug may influence the ability of the compound to control the symptoms in question.

Antiemetic (an-thai-em-et-ick)

A drug that prevents nausea. This may help with restoring fluid stores in the body, thus enhancing how well the body can handle its natural functions.

Anus (eh-nus)

The opening of the alimentary canal. The opening appears between the buttocks.

Appendicitis (ah-pen-di-sigh-tus)

Inflammation of the appendix. The condition may cause irritation and pain and could require the organ to be removed.

Appendix (ap-end-dicks)

A small extension that appears off the cecum. The organ is believed to help control the digestive system after a diarrheal condition develops, although it is unclear as to whether the appendix does anything. The appendix may be removed through a surgical procedure for the protection of the patient.

Ascites (as-sigh-ties)

The collection of fluid inside the peritoneal cavity.

Ascorbic Acid (as-soar-bick)

Also known as vitamin C. This is a water-soluble nutrient that may assist in clearing free radicals from the body. This may be administered in a supplement form if necessary, although it also appears naturally in citrus fruits and some vegetables.

Aspartame (as-par-tame)

An artificial sweetener made from aspartic acid and phenylalanine. This may be found in some food products that claim to be sugar-free.

Avitaminosis (eh-vee-at-min-oh-sis)

A disease that develops due to the body not getting enough of a certain vitamin. The disease may be referred to by the scientific name of a vitamin or the general letter or number name of that vitamin.

Bariatric Surgery (bear-e-a-trick)

A surgical procedure designed for those who are extremely overweight or obese. The goal is to reduce the patient's weight as soon as possible, thus reducing risks. Part of the procedure includes reducing the pocket of food storage in the body, thus potentially reducing the number of calories that a person is capable of consuming in one day. The procedure may be reversible or could fail depending on how well the body is able to handle the treatment involved.

Bariatrics (bear-e-a-trix)

Actions that focus on helping people who are obese. This may include surgery and other common processes needed for keeping a person's weight down.

Beriberi (berry-berry)

A deficiency in thiamin or vitamin B1. The condition develops as wet beriberi that may influence the heart and circulatory system. The issue may cause heart failure. Edema may also develop in some patients.

Bezoar (bez-oar)

Swallowed fibers, hair, and other items that may be found in the alimentary canal. These materials may have to be removed over time to control the digestive system and to prevent problems from occurring.

Bile (By-ul)

A fluid that is produced in the liver and stored in the gall bladder. The material will move into the duodenum. Bile assists in supporting the digestive function in the body.

The fluid is green or yellow in tone and is analyzed through a sample taken from the liver.

Biliary (bill-e-air-e)

Relating to the gall bladder, bile ducts, or bile fluid.

Bilirubin (bill-e-rue-bin)

An orange-yellow pigment found in bile. The pigment gives the bile its distinct color.

Biotin (by-oh-tin)

An enzyme co-factor found in living cells. The compound may be found in the kidney and liver rather than most other parts of the body. The vitamin triggers metabolic functions and is the way the body processes fats, amino acids, and carbohydrates. It is also called vitamin B7 or vitamin H.

Body Mass Index

Also known as BMI. A measure of the total body fat in an adult's body. The value is based on a person's height and weight. The BMI is a measure of the kilograms per square meter in the body. A person with a BMI from 18.5 to 25 is interpreted as being healthy. A person who has a BMI of 30 or greater may be identified as being obese.

Bolus (bowl-us)

A soft mass of food that has been chewed and is ready to be swallowed. The bolus should move through the digestive system and be broken down accordingly.

Borborygmus (bor-bore-ge-mus)

The process of belching. This is a sign that a person has taken in more gas in the body than can regularly be handled.

Botulism (bot-ue-li-zim)

A form of food poisoning caused by the Clostridium botulinum bacterium. The condition develops when a person consumed poisoned or improperly prepared food, although the condition may develop due to a wound infection. The condition is rare but may be fatal. This can cause muscle weakness if not treated properly.

Bowel Movement

Also known as defecation or as BM. A process at the end of the digestive cycle. The solid or liquid waste in the body will be eliminated through the anus. The process happens daily or a few times a week. Some people may have three bowel movements in a day, although three may happen in a week. Cases, where bowel movements are not produced regularly, may be a sign of certain medical issues that may negatively influence the body's functionality.

Bulimia (bul-ee-mee-ah)

An eating disorder where a person consumes a large amount of food in a brief period of time. This may be due to an unusual craving for various foods.

Bulimia Nervosa (nur-voe-sah)

A form of bulimia where a person binge eats, or quickly consumes a large amount of food, and then purges the food. This may involve a person intentionally vomiting and using laxatives. The concern is a mental disorder caused by a person trying to avoid gaining weight.

Cachexia (kach-ex-ee-ah)

Ill health that is associated with a chronic illness. A person may experience a lack of proper nutrition and could be at risk of losing weight.

Caffeine (caff-een)

An alkaloid drug found in tea, coffee, and various carbonated beverages. The drug will trigger functions in the central nervous system causing it to become more aware and alert. The drug may also trigger feelings of fatigue after it wears off. Caffeine produces a diuretic effect.

CAH

Chronic active hepatitis. A condition where a person has hepatitis for at least three months. The condition may be paired with events of cell necrosis and could involve the production of cirrhosis.

Calorie (kal-or-ee)

The energy the body requires to increase the temperature of a gram of water by one degree Celsius. This is the form of energy that may be consumed in the body through the treatment of fluids. An excess amount of calories in the body may result in weight gain due to the body being unable to burn off the weight.

Capsule Endoscope

An endoscope found in a small pill. The patient will swallow the capsule that contains the small camera. The unit will then move through the digestive system through the gastrointestinal tract. A wireless link will identify what the camera sees, thus allowing the doctor to identify the issues that have developed in the tissues. The endoscope should be naturally removed by the body through a bowel movement.

Carbohydrate

An organic compound also known as a carb. Starch, cellulose, glycogen, and polysaccharides are among the most common carbohydrates. A carb will provide a person with extra energy and can help facilitate many physical functions. An excess number of carbs may cause difficulties relating to how foods are processed and could result in weight gain.

Cardia (car-de-ah)

A part of the stomach near the opening from the esophagus to the stomach. The area gets its name because it is the closest part of the stomach to the heart.

Carotene (kare-oh-tin)

A red or yellow compound found in various vegetables, particularly in leafy vegetables, carrots, and sweet potatoes. Carotene may be found in various vitamin A-rich foods, although an excess consumed may cause difficulties in the body where the vitamin is not absorbed correctly.

Casein (case-een)

A milk protein. The compound includes various essential amino acids as well as some of the more common ones.

Cecum (see-kum)

The outward area of the large intestine that goes below the first part of the small intestine. This is the first section of the colon. The cecum has a worm-like appearance as it extends out from the rest of the tissue.

Celiac (see-lee-ack)

Relating to the abdominal opening inside the body.

Celiac Disease

An autoimmune disorder or gluten-sensitive enteropathy. The body produces an immune reaction to the consumption of gluten. The small intestine develops inflammation and can trigger bloating and diarrhea when the compound is consumed. The issue may also trigger malabsorption, a condition where the body is unable to absorb some nutrients.

Cellulose (cell-ue-lose)

An insoluble compound that produces plant cell walls and vegetable fibers. The material will influence how well the body functions.

Cholangitis (ko-lan-gie-tis)

Inflammation in the gallbladder.

Cholelithiasis (ko-le-lith-i-ah-sis)

The development of gallstones in the gallbladder.

Cholera (kol-ur-ah)

A bacterial disease that develops when a person consumes contaminated water. This may cause dehydration and diarrhea. The condition is not prominent in modern countries where sanitation is available. However, the condition can be deadly if it is contracted and is not treated with antibiotics and rehydration. The condition is found mainly in Southeast Asia and much of India.

Cholestasis (kol-e-stay-sis)

When bile flow is reduced. The condition may be caused by a blockage at the liver. The condition may trigger intense itching around the body and struggles with handling bowel movements. A liver infection or gallstones may be the cause. Patients with liver cancer are at high risk.

Chronic Ulcerative Colitis

Inflammation along the inside of the colon. The chronic condition may develop often in people who have Crohn's disease.

Chyle (kyle)

A white fluid that comes out of the small intestines and into the lymphatic system. The fluid includes lymph tissues and fat droplets. The chyle will drain during the digestive process.

Chylothorax (ky-lo-for-ax)

When chyle develops in the thorax. The fluid may build up in the area.

Cirrhosis (sur-hoe-sis)

A condition where the liver experiences degeneration. Liver cells are replaced with scar tissue. The condition develops due to alcohol abuse or chronic hepatitis. The organ will be unable to function properly. This may trigger fatigue and excess weight loss. Jaundice may also develop in some cases.

Colitis (col-eye-tis)

Inflammation in the colon. This may also be called ulcerative colitis or UC. The inflammation may prevent the colon from receiving blood. Inflammatory bowel disease or IBD may also develop. An excess total of white blood cells can be found in the region.

Colon (cole-in)

The large intestine. The tissue appears prior to the rectum. The organ removes water, salt, and various nutrients from the stool.

Colonoscopy (col-in-os-coe-pee)

An exam that uses an endoscope. The endoscope reviews the inside part of the colon to identify any polyps or other unusual tissues that may form. The ability of the endoscope to move through the intestine and colon may also be analyzed. The procedure is recommended among those who are at least 40 years of age.

Colorectal Cancer

A malignant growth in the large intestine. Also known as colon cancer. The issue develops from polyps. Patients who have benign polyps in the colon may be at an elevated risk of developing colorectal cancer later on.

Colostomy (col-os-toe-mee)

An opening in the large intestine. The term may also refer to the procedure needed to make the opening. The intestine will be brought out outside of the abdominal wall. One end will move through a cut in the abdominal wall, thus creating a stoma. A pouch that gathers fecal matter will be installed in the stoma. The procedure is for those who are unable to manage bowel movements on their own and require help in the process.

Constipation (con-stip-a-shun)

When a person is unable to have regular bowel movements. This may be triggered by a person not eating the fiber or other nutrients needed to support the development of a healthy bowel movement. Constipation may develop in cases where a person has fewer than three bowel movements in a week.

Corpulence (cor-pue-lince)

Obesity.

Craving

A desire to consume something. This may be an intense hunger for food. The issue may be triggered by hormones or by various types of stimuli.

Crohn's Disease (krones)

Also known as ileitis - inflammation that develops in the intestine. This frequent condition causes diarrhea and fatigue and may lead to weight loss and an inability to absorb nutrients properly. The condition may not appear in an impacted person for a while, but some chronic symptoms may be persistent.

Diarrhea (dye-ah-ree-ah)

An issue where a person experiences multiple loose bowel movements in one day. The movement may be excess liquid being cleared out of the body. A person who has at least three of these movements in one day may have diarrhea. The condition produces dehydration and abdominal pains.

Dietary Fiber

A carbohydrate that is not digestible through the body's enzymes. Fiber is found in various fruits, vegetables, and grains. The compound may help with adding bulk to bowel movements.

Digestion

A process where the body will convert foods into substances that can be absorbed by the body. The substances have to be broken down for metabolic activities and to allow the body to stay nourished. Various enzymes in the body are responsible for ensuring the digestive process continues normally.

Digital Rectal Exam

A test also referred to as a DRE. The exam analyzes the quality of the prostate. The doctor will insert a lubricated and gloved finger into the rectum to analyze the area. The test is used to identify prostate cancer in men.

Diverticulitis (dye-ver-tick-ue-lye-tis)

Inflammation in the diverticula.

Diverticulosis (di-ver-tick-ue-loe-sis)

The appearance of many diverticula. These pouches will appear in the colonic wall.

Diverticulum (di-ver-tick-ue-lum)

A pouch that develops in a saccular organ. This may be found in the gastrointestinal tract. The sac occurs around a weak spot in the wall along the tract. The condition may form while straining during a bowel movement, a concern that especially develops in the large intestine. The large intestine is more likely to develop the diverticulum.

Duodenitis (duo-den-eye-tis)

Inflammation in the duodenum in the small intestine.

Duodenum (duo-den-um)

The first part of the small intestine. The tissue connects the pylorus to the jejunum.

Dysentery (dis-en-tear-e)

An intestinal infection that causes diarrhea. The issue is caused by the consumption of contaminated water or food. The shigellosis bacteria will trigger the development. People in Southeast Asia and India are more likely to develop dysentery than other areas where proper sanitation is available. Bloody diarrhea may develop when the issue occurs.

Dyspepsia (dis-pep-see-ah)

Difficulties with digesting foods. The problem develops after eating. The digestive tract becomes inflamed.

Dysphagia (dis-fay-jah)

A condition where a person is unable to swallow properly. The condition may be oropharyngeal, which means the person is unable to start swallowing the food. Esophageal dysphagia will occur when a person feels that the food one is stuck in the neck or chest and is not being processed properly.

EGD

Esophagogastroduodenoscopy - a process that uses an endoscope to identify issues in the upper gastrointestinal tract. The analysis reviews how the area is treated and if there are blockages or unusual growths. The process will include a review of the esophagus, stomach, and small intestine.

Epidermal Growth Factor

Also called EGF. The factor triggers the growth of cells and how they are differentiated. The EGF binds to a receptor and may work with different amino acids to process the body's functions.

Electrolyte (e-leck-tro-lite)

A compound that splits into multiple ions and then creates an electric charge in the body. The electrolyte is found in some fluids that one consumes, particularly sports drinks.

Elimination

A process where a person removes wastes from one's body. This is another term for a bowel movement.

Emetics (em-et-icks)

A concern that relates to patient vomiting. This may be noted through the suffix – emesis.

Encopresis (en-coe-pree-sis)

When a person is unable to control their bowel movement. A doctor may diagnose the condition if a child is four years old or older. The concern may involve swelling in the bowels, thus keeping a person from being able to have bowel movements without obstruction.

Enema (en-im-ah)

A drug that enters the rectum to clear the colon. The enema is often applied in order to do diagnostic testing processes to ensure no parts of the bowels are in the way. The enema works after a person consumes a liquid diet and laxatives for 24 hours prior to the diagnostic test. The enema tube is then inserted in the rectum with barium sulfate and water being flushed into the colon. An x-ray is taken of the area. The barium solution is then drained through the tube after the test is completed.

Enteritis (en-tur-eye-tis)

Inflammation in the small intestine. Any part of the organ may be influenced.

Enterocolitis (en-tur-kole-eye-tis)

Inflammation in the membranes in both the small and large intestines.

Enterocytes (en-tur-oh-sites)

Cells in the small intestine that support the digestion and absorption of nutrients and other compounds.

Enterostomy (en-tur-aws-toe-mee)

A surgical procedure where the small intestine is adjusted to move to a new opening formed in another segment of the intestine or in the abdominal wall. The process is used when the tissue has been negatively influenced and a portion of the intestine has to be removed.

Epiglottis (ep-eh-glot-tis)

The cartilage that covers the windpipe like a lid that keeps food from entering the trachea.

Epulis (ep-o-lis)

Swelling on the gum - a tumor may form on the gingival mucosa.

ERCP

Endoscopic retrograde cholangiopancreatogram. The test uses endoscopic and fluoroscopic procedures to identify how bile ducts function. Any unusual qualities found in the tissue may be diagnosed in the testing process.

Esophageal Achalasia (es-oh-fa-jeel ach-al-ay-sha)

The inability of the lower esophageal sphincter to relax. The stress prevents the esophagus from functioning accordingly.

Esophageal Varices (vair-eh-cees)

When the esophagus has or develops wider veins. The condition may cause intense bleeding. People who abuse alcohol have a high risk of developing the issue.

Esophagitis (es-oh-faj-eye-tis)

Inflammation in the esophagus.

Esophagus (es-ah-fa-gus)

A passage between the stomach and pharynx. This is located in the gastrointestinal tract and supports how foods and liquids enter and are processed in the body.

Eustachian Tube (you-stay-shin)

A canal found from the middle ear to the pharynx.

Feces (fee-cees)

Excrement that is produced through the intestines. The compound includes unabsorbed solids and waste products in the body along with some harmful forms of bacteria. It is also called fecal matter. The removal of feces is necessary to ensure the body can clear waste materials.

Flatulence (flat-u-lince)

The production of gas in the gastrointestinal tract. The gas is expelled through the anus. The gas may be the product of the tract's ability to break down foods.

Gallbladder (gall-blad-ur)

A small organ in the body near the small intestine and beneath the liver. Bile is gathered in the organ. The compound is then released into the small intestine. The gallbladder is necessary to ensure bile is handled appropriately.

Gallstone (gall-stone)

A mass that develops in the biliary tract including in the gallbladder. The stone is hardened and may develop a yellow color. The material may include cholesterol that has not dissolved, although some other components from inside the body may be a part of the tissue. The gallstone may be naturally removed from the body, although this may produce intense pain. If pain persists or becomes worse, an operation to remove the stone may be necessary.

Gastralgia (gas-tral-gee-ah)

Pains in the stomach or abdomen.

Gastrectomy (gas-treck-toe-mee)

The removal of part or all of the stomach. The intestine may have to be rerouted if the stomach has to be completely removed. The procedure is to deal with stomach cancer in most cases.

Gastric (gas-trick)

Relating to the stomach.

Gastric Absorption

The process where the stomach takes in various substances.

Gastritis (gas-try-tis)

Inflammation of the lining of the stomach.

Gastroenteritis (gas-tro-en-tur-eye-tis)

Inflammation in the gastrointestinal tract.

Gastroesophageal Reflux Disease

Also known as GERD. A condition that impacts the lower esophageal sphincter in the stomach. The tissue is a ring of muscle that links the esophagus to the stomach. The condition is chronic and may result in stomach acid and bile flowing into the food pipe. The condition will cause the lining to be irritated. The condition may be diagnosed if the condition occurs at least twice a week with acid reflux and heartburn.

Gastrointestinal Tract (gas-tro-in-tes-tin-ul)

The digestive structures that go from the mouth to the anus. This does not involve the liver, pancreas, or biliary tract. It may be called the GI tract for short.

Gastroparesis (gas-tro-par-ee-sis)

When the gastric system does not empty properly. This may be a chronic concern.

Gastrostomy (gas-tro-stoe-mee)

A surgical procedure where an outside opening is produced in the stomach. An opening is produced through the abdominal wall. A tube is applied to allow food to enter into the stomach, thus facilitating the natural process of breaking down and taking in nutrients. The process is for cases where swallowing is difficult or the nutrients one requires consistently break down before they can be introduced into the body the right way.

Gavage (ga-vah-ge)

The administration of food or drugs into the body by force. The process may particularly be used when taking care of an animal's health. The administration uses a tube that goes down the throat and into the stomach.

Gingivitis (gin-ge-veye-tis)

Inflammation of the gums. The inflammation develops when a person engages in inappropriate oral hygiene. The condition can trigger irritation and redness in the gums. Swelling may also develop in the area. The problem can result in tooth decay and loss if not treated properly. The gums may also bleed in some cases.

Gleason Score

A score that identifies the health of the male prostate and a tumor in the area during a test. The score may be from 6 to 10. A lower score suggests that there are no substantial issues with the tumor and that it is not overly aggressive, thus suggesting that cancer may be treated. When the score is high, the tumor may be likely to spread and create significant problems in the body if not handled.

Glossitis (gloss-eye-tis)

Inflammation in the tongue.

Glycemic Index

A numerical review that will monitor the blood glucose rate. A high GI number may indicate the increase of blood glucose levels that may require medication or diet to control. A low GI number indicates the body is digesting carbs and releasing them slowly, which allows energy levels to be sustained appropriately.

Glycemic Load

A value of the food that one consumes that is equal to the glycemic index of the food multiplied by the carbohydrate content within that food.

Glycine (gl-eye-seen)

An amino acid that makes up fibroin and gelatin which is considered a nutrient.

Heartburn

A burning sensation in the chest. The sensation occurs when a person experiences gastric juice moving back into the esophagus.

Hematemesis (hee-mah-tem-eh-sis)

An emergency condition where a person vomits blood. The body may experience some irritation.

Hemorrhoids (hemo-or-oids)

Veins swelling along the bottom part of the anus and rectum. The veins stretch and bulge and become painful. The condition may become worse when the person defecates. The inflammation can cause intense swelling. The veins will swell due to straining during bowel movements. Those who are overweight and pregnant women are more likely to develop hemorrhoids.

Hepatic (hep-ah-tick)

Relating to the liver.

Hepatitis (hep-ah-tie-tis)

Inflammation of the liver. The condition may trigger cirrhosis in some cases. There are four types of hepatitis infections that are triggered by different causes and may produce varying side effects.

Hepatitis A (hep-at-eye-tis)

A liver infection triggered by the hepatitis virus. The condition spreads from infected food or water. This may cause flu-like symptoms and jaundice. The condition may be prevented by an appropriate vaccine.

Hepatitis B

An infection that develops in the liver after being caused by the hepatitis virus. The condition may be prevented by a vaccine. The condition may be inflammation in the liver, although it can evolve into cirrhosis in the late stage. A person may contract HepB through exposure to infected body compounds.

Hepatitis C

A form of the hepatitis virus that is spread through contact with contaminated blood. This may happen when people share needles. If a person is in contact with unsterile tattoo equipment while getting a tattoo on the skin may also trigger HepC. The virus may not produce symptoms in all cases, although those with the issue may develop a loss of appetite and sudden nausea.

Hepatitis D

A liver condition that develops in the body of a person who has the Hepatitis B virus. HepD occurs when the HepB virus requires extra help for managing the replication process. People who regularly abuse intravenous drugs and those who have had many blood transfusions will be at a high risk of developing this issue.

Hepatoblastoma (hep-ah-toe-blas-toe-mah)

A cancerous tumor that develops in the liver. It develops mainly among children, although it could occur at any age. The tumor occurs in the right lobe in most cases.

Hepatocyte (hep-ah-toe-cite)

Liver cells. The cells produce many of the metabolic and secretory functions that develop in the body.

Hepatoma (hep-ah-toe-mah)

A malignant tumor in the liver. This is a common type of liver cancer. Patients who abuse alcohol are more likely to develop hepatoma.

Hepatomegaly (hep-ah-toe-may-gal-ee)

When the liver becomes enlarged. Bloating in the abdominal area may develop. The change in the liver may be a sign of more significant concern, particularly cirrhosis.

Herpes Labialis (hur-pees lay-bee-al-is)

Cold sores produced by the herpes simplex I virus.

Hyperemesis Gravidarum (grav-eh-dar-um)

Vomiting that occurs during the early part of pregnancy. This may be more intense than the normal morning sickness that occurs at the start of a pregnancy. A woman will require IV fluids and anti-nausea treatment drugs to control the condition.

Hyperphagia (high-pur-phay-ge-ah)

Overeating.

IBW

Ideal body weight. This is used when a person is at least 60 inches in height and is an approximation for what a person should expect. For men, the IBW is calculated by 50 kg multiplied by one's height in inches minus 60. For women, the IBW is calculated by 45.5 kg multiplied by one's height in inches minus 60.

Inflammatory Bowel Disease

Also known as IBD. The inflammation develops in the digestive tract. The entire tract may be influenced. Ulcerative colitis and Crohn's disease are the most common IBDs.

Irritable Bowel Syndrome

Also known as IBS. The syndrome impacts the large intestine. Abdominal cramping and bloating can develop. Constipation may also develop. The cause is unclear, but a diagnosis may be made based on the symptoms the patient expresses.

Ileectomy (il-e-eck-toe-mee)

The removal of the ileum.

Ileitis (il-ee-eye-tis)

Inflammation in the ileum.

Ileostomy (il-eh-os-toe-mee)

A procedure where an opening for the ileum appears on the abdominal wall.

Ileum (il-ee-um)

The narrow part of the small intestine. This is a tissue that appears between the jejunum and ileocecal valve in the large intestine.

Ileus (il-e-us)

When the flow of the contents in the intestine are unable to make it through the bowel.

Intestines (in-tess-tins)

The segments in the digestive system that processes food from the stomach into the anal canal. The organs will move wastes through and filter out the nutrients that need to remain in the body. Proper functioning of the intestines is needed to ensure good health.

Intussusception (in-tuss-u-cept-shun)

A process where the intestine moves into its body. A portion of the intestine will contract into the nearby lumen. The condition causes bowel obstruction as the passageway starts to narrow. Children are more likely to develop the issue than others. The trouble may be fatal if not treated properly. An enema may help push the intestine back in its place. Surgery may be required if the enema does not work.

Inulin (in-ue-lin)

Starch in the roots of various plants. The compound identifies how well a kidney may function. High amounts could be administered so that the kidneys can be tested to see how well they will respond to these materials.

Jaundice (jon-dis)

A condition where the skin and eyes become yellow. This is due to bilirubin building up within the body. The liver will be unable to process the compound, thus leading to jaundice. This may develop in those who regularly consume alcohol, although a newborn whose liver is not fully developed upon birth may also deal with the condition.

Jejunal (jay-jue-nul)

Relating to the jejunum.

Jejunum (jay-jue-num)

A part of the small intestine that links the duodenum to the ileum. This is the second part of the small intestine.

Labial Mucosa (lay-be-ul mue-coe-sah)

The inside lining in the lips.

Lactase (lack-tase)

An enzyme that supports the hydrolysis of lactose to glucose and galactose. Lactase is required to help the body handle lactose. Those who are unable to tolerate lactase may struggle when consuming dairy products.

Lactic Acid

An acid produced through the fermentation of carbohydrates found in dairy products, particularly milk. The acid is produced when the body does not have enough oxygen needed to handle the process to break down glucose for energy purposes.

Lactose (lack-tose)

Sugar in milk that includes molecules of glucose and galactose. A person who is unable to process the lactose sugar will be unable to handle dairy products without experiencing intense gastric distress. Lactase supplementation may be required to help the body to be capable of consuming lactose materials.

Laxative

A compound that softens the material in the bowels. A medicated agent will soften the stool and keep the bowels from being bound. A laxative helps relieve constipation.

Leukoplakia (lou-koe-plak-ee-ah)

A white patch found on a mucous membrane. The patch is imbedded inside the mouth and is not able to be removed. The condition is noncancerous, although it may be a sign of a person is more likely to contract a cancerous condition. The patch is also known as smoker's keratosis.

Lingual (lin-gual)

Relating to the tongue.

Lipolysis (lip-ol-eh-sis)

The body's process of metabolizing fat.

Liver Function Test

A test to identify how the liver responses to damages. Tests are conducted to determine how well the liver creates albumin and bilirubin. The tests for the two compounds are produced separately from one another. Blood is gathered from the liver to identify the two compounds. If the body does not have enough of these materials, it has to be remedied by a physician.

Lysine (ly-seen)

An essential amino acid. The compound builds protein for muscle mass. Lysine may also be used as a medication for treating cold sores triggered by the herpes simplex labialis virus.

Malabsorption (mal-ab-sore-p-shun)

When the body is unable to absorb nutrients appropriately.

Malnutrition

When the body is unable to take in the nutrients it requires.

Mastication (mas-tick-ay-shun)

The process of chewing food.

Megacolon

When the colon becomes larger than necessary. The immense dilation may keep the bowel from being fully functional.

Melena (mel-en-ah)

A black stool that appears due to upper gastrointestinal bleeding. The blood has been damaged heavily by intestinal enzymes. The condition may develop due to the stomach having at least 50 mL of blood. The condition may cause the stool to look unusual for a few days with the first stool appearing a few hours after the blood is first ingested by the stomach.

Mesenteric (mes-en-tur-ick)

Involving the double layer of peritoneum that keeps the intestine away from the back part of the abdominal wall.

Mesentery (mes-en-tair-ee)

A double layer of peritoneum. The tissue will keep the intestines in place while staying along the back area of the abdominal wall without being in direct contact with the tissue.

Mucositis (mew-coe-sigh-tis)

Inflammation in a mucous membrane. Such membranes appear mainly in the mouth and throat areas.

Nasogastric (nay-so-gas-trick)

A material that is provided to the body by using a tube that is inserted through the nose. The compound that is administered in the procedure will go through into the stomach.

Nausea (naw-zha)

A feeling in the stomach that produces discomfort. The person may be at a high risk of vomiting.

Norovirus (nor-oh-vie-rus)

A virus associated with gastroenteritis.

Obesity (oh-bee-sit-ee)

When a person is greatly overweight. Excess subcutaneous fat develops under the skin and visceral fat builds up around the organs. Obesity develops when a person's body mass index or BMI is at least 30. A person who is obese will be at an elevated risk of developing significant medical issues including diabetes and heart-related concerns.

Obstipation (ob-stip-ay-shun)

Constipation that develops and lasts for a while. A person will have three or fewer bowel movements in a week. Any stool that is produced will be hard or dry in texture. Constipation occurs because there is a blockage in the intestines. A procedure is required for clearing the intestines; this may require an endoscope.

Odynophagia (oh-de-no-fay-jah)

Pains when swallowing. Swallowing difficulties can occur.

Omentum (oh-men-tum)

A peritoneum fold that connects to the stomach and other organs around the abdominal cavity. The tissue covers the liver, intestine, and stomach.

Oropharynx (or-oh-fair-inx)

A middle part of the pharynx. The area lies behind the mouth and near the soft palate and is known as the throat. The tissue is responsible for the swallowing process and for getting food to move from the mouth to the esophagus.

Ostomy (os-toe-mee)

A surgical procedure to create an opening or stoma in a part of the body. For the digestive system, the treatment produces an artificial opening in the GI canal.

Pancreas (pan-cree-as)

A gland behind the stomach. The pancreas produces a juice that enters the intestine to support regular digestive functions and the body's ability to process nutrients. The organ also produces insulin, glucagon, and somatostatin to enter the bloodstream. A person who has diabetes might not have a pancreas that is fully operational or active.

Pancreatectomy

The removal of the pancreas through surgery. The treatment is to control chronic pancreatitis in cases where other treatment methods have not worked to control the situation. The person would require added medications that include artificial insulin injections and digestive enzymes to handle the functions that are no longer being provided by the regular pancreas tissue.

Parotid Gland

A salivary gland found in many bodies. There are two of these glands on the sides of the mouth and in front of the ears.

Parotitis (pear-oh-tie-tis)

Inflammation in the parotid gland.

Pecten (pec-tin)

The narrow spot in the anal canal located in the middle section.

PEG

Percutaneous endoscopic gastrostomy. The procedure involves passing a tube into the patient's stomach through the abdominal wall. The process provides a consistent means of feeding in cases where a person cannot take food orally.

Pellagra (pel-ag-rah)

A disease that develops due to a lack of niacin or vitamin B3. The condition may cause dermatitis, diarrhea, and dementia, and can be fatal if not treated.

Peptic Ulcer

An ulcer that develops in the gastrointestinal tract. The ulcer may happen when the tract in contact with gastric juice for too long. The condition may cause intense pains.

Perihepatitis (pear-ee-hep -a-tie-tis)

Inflammation in the peritoneal cavity in the liver.

Peristalsis (pear-e-stawl-sis)

A movement in the body that is triggered by sudden muscle contraction. The action will cause the contents of the intestines or other organs in the body to move in one direction.

Peritoneal Absorption

The uptake of materials in the peritoneal cavity.

Peritoneal Cavity (pear-e-tone-eel)

An area that is secured by the peritoneum. The cavity is found in the liver between two sacs. These sacs are found behind the stomach and are connected to one another through the epiploic foramen.

Polyp (pol-ip)

A tissue mass that sticks to the lumen in the digestive tract. The tissue growth occurs from a mucous membrane and may be pedunculated if it is linked to a surface through a narrow stalk or sessile. If there are no stalks, it links directly to the inside of the tract. A polyp may be found in the stomach, nose, bladder, or uterus among other areas, although it is most likely to be found in the colon. A polyp is benign and may cause an obstruction in some cases. The issue may also be a predictor of colon cancer in some patients.

Portal Vein

A vein that transports blood from the digestive organs and other parts of the body to the liver.

Postprandial (post-pran-dee-al)

After a meal.

Prebiotics (pre-by-ot-ix)

Ingredients in foods that will support the development of probiotic bacteria in the large intestine. The ingredients are indigestible and will influence how the body produces healthy tissues.

Proctocolitis (prock-toe-coe-lie-tis)

Inflammation in the colon.

Proctoscope

An endoscope that is inserted in the rectum and anus to inspect these tissues.

Proteolysis (pro-tee-oh-ly-sis)

When proteins break down into peptides and amino acids. Enzymes in the digestive tract will help support the process.

PUD

Peptic ulcer disease. The condition is caused by sores or ulcers that develop in the lining in the stomach or the opening area in the small intestine. The stomach ulcer will cause abdominal pain. The overuse of anti-inflammatory pain relievers like aspirin and the development of the H. Pylori bacteria will cause the issue, although the ability of the ulcer to develop may be random depending on the patient.

Pylorus (py-lore-us)

A section in the stomach that has an opening between the stomach and duodenum.

Pyrosis (py-roe-sis)

A burning sensation in the body. The pain may e caused by gastric juice moving back up the esophagus by regurgitation. The condition is also called heartburn.

RDA

The recommended daily allowance of a nutrient. The RDA varies based on the person's physical demands, any conditions that a person has, and the type of nutrient that is required for general health.

Rectum (wreck-tum)

A distal part of the large intestine. This is the last part of the organ. The rectum ends at the anus and supports the body's ability to clear out waste.

Retention

How the body can hold its fluids and foods. A body that can retain these foods will be likely to support the nutrients it requires for general health.

Saliva (sal-eye-vah)

A fluid that is produced by the salivary glands in the mouth. The fluid is naturally generated to keep the oral area moist and to support the digestion of starches. A lack of saliva may keep a patient from being able to chew, swallow, and break down foods properly. The dry mouth resulting from not having saliva may also influence a person's breath and could damage the teeth.

Salivary Ducts

Ducts that transport saliva.

Salivary Glands

Glands that produce the saliva in the mouth. These include the parotid gland in the back part of the mouth, the submandibular gland around the bottom part, and the sublingual gland near the central region in the mouth.

Salmonella (sal-min-el-ah)

An infection triggered by the salmonella bacteria. The condition occurs when a person consumes contaminated food or water. Unwashed produce, raw meat, and raw eggs are more likely to trigger salmonella conditions. People who directly handle reptiles may also contract the bacteria. The condition can trigger abdominal pains, chills, and diarrhea, although those symptoms are more significant among those with immune system difficulties.

Small Bowel

Also known as the small intestine or SB. This is where much of the body's absorption of food takes place. The tissue includes the duodenum, jejunum, and ileum. The tissue is about an inch in diameter and could be up to twenty feet long.

Small Bowel Obstruction

When a polyp, clot, blockage, or another type of obstruction develops in the small intestine or bowel. Also called SBO.

Scurvy (skur-vee)

A blood vessel condition that develops due to the body not having enough vitamin C or ascorbic acid. The condition causes bleeding in the skin and gums and may produce a soft feeling in the gums. The body may also become exceptionally worn and weak if scurvy is present.

Sialadenitis (see-al-ad-en-eye-tis)

Inflammation in a salivary gland.

Sialorrhea (see-al-or-ea)

An excessive amount of salivary flow. This may be triggered by the salivary glands functioning improperly. A tumor may be found on one of the glands.

Sigmoid (sig-moid)

The last part of the large intestine, the sigmoid lead to the rectum. The sigmoid is noted for having an S-shape.

Stoma (stoe-mah)

An opening that is produced in the body. A stoma may be natural as one organ in the digestive system attaches to another, but the stoma may also be artificially produced. This would require a tube being inserted in one part of the body while linking to the organ in question. The process of creating a new stoma is for cases where the body is unable to handle certain functions on its own. The process of creating the stoma may be risky.

Stomach

A digestive organ in the upper left part of the abdomen and appears in between the esophagus and duodenum. The stomach takes in the foods that go through the esophagus and will store and digests them. The materials that are broken down will then move through the duodenum so they are prepared to be eliminated from the body.

Stomach Ulcer

An ulcer that develops on the inside part of the stomach tissue. The ulcer may stick directly to the gastric mucosa or be hanging off a small thread material. The ulcer will develop due to the stomach being in contact with intense gastric juice.

Stomatitis (stow-mah-tie-tis)

Inflammation within the soft parts of the mouth. The inflammation may include a sore.

Stool

Fecal matter expelled through the anus. The compound moves out through the anus from the intestines.

Sublingual Gland (sub-lin-gual)

The salivary gland under the tongue.

Sucrose (sue-crows)

A form of sugar. The material comes from sugar beets or sugar cane. The sugar may directly influence blood levels.

Supraglottitis (sue-pra-glot-ty-tis)

Inflammation in the larynx or the windpipe that appears before the voice box. The condition may be caused by bacteria, although the influenza virus and strep infections are most common. The issue may be life-threatening as it may influence the ability of a person to breathe properly.

Tenesmus (ten-es-mis)

A condition where a person is unable to fully clear their bowel when defecating. The patient may feel they are unable to clear the large bowel even if that person has nothing left to clear. The issue will trigger intense pains and cramping among other digestive indications.

Tongue

An organ in the mouth. The pink body features a mucosa compound with small bumps called papillae. The tissue includes the taste buds needed to enjoy food. The tongue also supports the development of saliva. The tongue is necessary for chewing and swallowing foods and for speech.

TPN

Total parenteral nutrition. The process involves feeding while moving food past the gastrointestinal tract. A formula that includes the nutrients the body requires is applied through a vein. The TPN allows the food to move through the target vein to the gastrointestinal system so the compound can be absorbed by the stomach and eventually processed by the body.

Trismus (tris-mis)

The inability of a person to open their mouth all the way. The muscles needed for this will develop a reduced range of motion.

Typhilitis

Inflammation in the cecum.

Typhoid Fever (tie-foyd)

Bacterial infection also called enteric fever. Typhoid fever develops when the Salmonella Typhi bacteria enters the blood and intestines. The fever occurs when a person eats or drinks food that has been contaminated, particularly by the fecal matter of someone who is infected. The body may develop a fever and general weakness. The condition is more common in less-developed parts of the world. Vaccination is recommended to any person planning to travel to a part of the world where the fever issue is common.

Uvula (ue-vu-la)

A small extension located at the back part of the soft palate. This may be noticed as a small dangling tissue. The uvula works with the soft palate to close off the nasopharynx when the mouth is closed. The closure ensures that food does not enter the nasal cavity. A failure in the uvula may cause food to move into the nasal cavity.

Vomit (vom-et)

When the contents in the stomach are forced through the mouth. The vomiting episode may develop due to a bacterial infection or another form of poisoning in the stomach. Vomiting may also be forced through medication or other physical action, particularly in cases where a person has ingested any kind of poisonous material.

Weaning

When the mother's milk is replaced with other food. The child may be weaned off the mother's milk after a certain length of time to prepare to consume other foods. The weaning process ensures the child is independent of the mother and supports the developing growth that the child needs.

Whey (way)

Liquid materials in milk after the casein, fat, and other fat-soluble compounds are removed from the fluid.

Important Prefixes

bil/i	bile or relating to the gallbladder
bucco/o	cheek
calor/I	heat
cec/o	cecum
celi/o	abdomen
cheil/o	lips
chol/e	gall tissue
cholangi/o	bile vessel
cholecyst/o	gallbladder
choledoch/o	bile duct
cirrh/o	orange in appearance
col/o	colon
colon/o	colon
dent/I	teeth
duoden/o	duodenum
enter/o	small intestine
epiglott/o	epiglottis
gastr/o	stomach

gingiv/o	gums
gloss/o	tongue
hel/c	ulcer
hepat/o	liver
ile/o	ileum
inguin/o	groin
jejun/o	jejunum
labi/o	labia
lapar/o	abdominal wall
lingu/o	tongue
odont/o	tooth
or/o	mouth
ori	mouth
palat/o	palate
proct/o	anus and rectum
ptyal/o	saliva
pylor/o	pylorus
rect/o	rectum
sial/o	saliva
sialaden/o	salivary gland
sigmold/o	sigmoid colon
stom/o	mouth
zymo	fermentation

Chapter 3 – Endocrine System

The endocrine system is a series of glands that release hormones into the body. The hormones are secreted by the glands and assist in controlling various functions. The system is subject to various tumors and other irregularities that may negatively influence the production of hormones and other compounds in the body. Some of the glands may be removed as a means of treating significant concerns in the body. However, replacement medications would be required for the patient's lifetime to offset any losses that develop due to those hormones no longer being produced regularly and naturally.

Adrenal Cortex

A body situated near the adrenal gland. The cortex controls how well the body responds to stress. This includes the production of hormones like cortisol and aldosterone.

Acromegaly (ak-roe-mee-gal-ee)

A condition where the pituitary gland produces an excess amount of growth hormone. This may cause some concerns where the patient's body is growing faster than is normal. This includes possible growth that may develop after puberty.

ACTH

Adrenocorticotropic hormone. This is a compound that is released by the anterior pituitary gland and may respond to various physical stresses in the body.

ADH

Antidiuretic hormone. A hormone needed to maintain blood pressure and water content. The hormone controls how much water the person has in their body and ensures the person does not urinate more than necessary.

Adrenalectomy (ad-reen-a-leck-toe-mee)

The removal of an adrenal gland through surgery. This may be done to remove either or both of the glands.

Adrenalitis (ad-ren-al-eye-tis)

Inflammation in the adrenal gland.

Albuminuria (al-bu-min-ur-ee-ah)

Albumin located in the urine. This suggests that the kidney may develop a form of disease.

Aldosterone (al-doe-stur-own)

A hormone produced by the adrenal cortex to allow the kidneys to control electrolyte levels and water balance.

Aldosteronism (al-doe-stur-own-ism)

When the adrenal glands produce more aldosterone than necessary.

Allopurinol (al-oh-purr-i-nol)

A compound that reduces the production of uric acid by controlling the development of xanthine oxidase. The medication is designed to control gout and kidney stones.

Antidiabetic

A drug that reduces the effects of diabetes mellitus.

Antidiuretic Hormone

A hormone that is produced in the hypothalamus and then enters the pituitary gland. The hormone controls how much water is removed in the body's urine.

AODM

Adult-onset diabetes mellitus. The condition develops as an adult due to factors like weight gain or an unhealthy lifestyle in general.

Bacteriuria (bac-tier-ee-ur-ee-ah)

The development of bacteria in the urine.

Blood Glucose

A measure of glucose in the blood measured in a diabetic patient's body. It is also called blood sugar.

Calcitonin (cal-cit-toe-nin)

A hormone produced by the thyroid gland to assist in controlling calcium levels in the blood.

Conn Syndrome

A concern where excess aldosterone is produced within the adrenal gland.

Cortisol (core-ti-sole)

A stress hormone.

Cretinism (cree-tin-izm)

A condition that develops due to a lack of thyroid hormone. The condition is congenital.

Diabetes Insipidus (in-sip-id-us)

A condition where the patient experiences excess urination. This may be due to the body not controlling its antidiuretic hormone properly.

Diabetes Mellitus (mell-eye-tus)

A condition that impacts the body's ability to handle glucose. This may be interpreted in Type I and II diabetes. Type I refers to when the body does not have enough insulin. Type II is when the body resists the insulin that it produces.

Diabetic Retinopathy (ret-in-oh-pah-thee)

An eye disease that impacts those who suffer from diabetes. The condition causes blood vessels in the retina to be damaged. This may result in blindness.

DKA

Diabetic ketoacidosis. The condition develops in those who have diabetes. The body produces excess ketones or blood acids. The extra glucose that develops in the body is not handled by the body properly, thus causing various ketoacids to develop and form around the body.

Electrolyte (elek-troh-lite)

A mineral found in the blood or another fluid in the body. The compound includes a slight electrical charge. The compound assists in keeping a person hydrated and may be found in various energy drinks, although it could be provided as a medication for people with significant concerns.

Epinephrine (e-pin-ef-rin)

A hormone known as adrenaline. The hormone is generated in the medulla of the adrenal gland. Epinephrine influences a person's ability to act during high-intensity situations or stressful events.

Estrogen (ess-troh-gin)

A hormone that is produced in the female body, although it may be found in the male body in small doses. The hormone encourages the reproductive development of the female body.

Exophthalmos (ecks-oh-fal-mose)

A bulging eyeball or eyeball that appears to be a little further out of its socket than normal. The condition is linked mainly to hyperthyroidism.

Fasting Blood Sugar

A measure of what the body's blood sugar is like when that person has not consumed anything recently or has been resting. The FBS may be less than 100 mg/dL or 5.6 mmol/L in most cases. Anything that is higher than this may suggest a person could be at risk of developing diabetes. A person who has an FBS of 126 mg/dL or 7 mmol/L or greater on two tests will be diagnosed as having diabetes.

Follicle-Stimulating Hormone

A hormone from the pituitary gland that will control how reproductive functions develop in the body. This may also help with controlling how hair grows. A lack of FSH may cause difficulties surrounding the body's ability to grow hair.

Growth Hormone

Also known as somatotropin – a growth hormone or GH is a peptide hormone that triggers the production of cells in the body. This includes the reproduction and regeneration of cells, thus helping to trigger the proper growth of the human body.

Gigantism (j-eye-gant-izm)

A condition where a child experiences excess growth hormone. The issue results in an unusual growth pattern.

Glucagon (glue-ka-gone)

A hormone produced within the pancreas to control the insulin development in the body.

Glucose (glue-cose)

A form of sugar found in the blood. Glucose provides energy to the cells. An excess amount may result in significant problems.

Glucose Tolerance Test

A test used to determine if a person has diabetes. A fasting glucose test identifies a person's natural blood sugar. A glucose solution is then consumed by the patient. Another glucose test is then conducted. The process identifies if the patient is experiencing significant problems handling glucose.

GnRH

Gonadotropin-releasing hormone. The hormone is released in the anterior pituitary gland and triggers the development of a follicle-stimulating hormone and luteinizing hormone.

Goiter (goy-tur)

A swelling that develops around the front of the neck. The thyroid gland is enlarged. The condition may indicate difficulties in the gland's ability to release hormones correctly.

Graves Disease

An immune disorder that prevents the thyroid gland from functioning.

Gynecomastia (geye-ne-coe-mas-tee-ah)

The swelling of breast tissue in the male body. This is caused by a hormonal imbalance. The condition is benign, although it can cause males to develop female breasts.

HCG

Human chorionic gonadotropin. A hormone that is developed in the placenta after it is implanted in the body during pregnancy. The hormone may be identified in a pregnancy test to confirm that a woman is pregnant. HCG may also be used in some diets to help burn off fat, although that would require an extremely low-calorie diet for the process to work properly.

HGF

Hepatocyte growth factor. This is a compound that influences how the body grows.

Hypercalcemia (high-pur-cal-cee-me-ah)

A condition where the blood has an excess amount of calcium.

Hyperglycemia (high-pur-gl-eye-cee-me-ah)

When the body has an excess amount of glucose and results in high blood sugar content, which is dangerous for diabetics.

Hyperinsulinism (high-pur-in-sul-in-izm)

When the blood has a high amount of insulin.

Hyperpituitarism (high-pur-pit-oo-it-tear-izm)

When the pituitary gland produces an excess amount of hormone.

Hyperthyroidism (high-purth-eye-roid-izm)

A condition where the thyroid gland produces an excess amount of hormones.

Hyperthyroxinemia (high-pur-thy-rocks-in-em-ee-ah)

An elevated amount of thyroxine in the blood.

Hypoglycemia (high-poe-gly-cee-mee-ah)

When the body has a low blood sugar or glucose level. This may be noted when the level is less than 70 mg/dL.

Impaired Glucose Tolerance

Also known as prediabetes. The condition occurs when a person has high blood sugar but it is not at the point where one might have diabetes. The condition may not exhibit any symptoms in some patients.

Insulin

A hormone produced within the pancreas. The compound controls glucose levels.

Insulinoma (in-sue-lin-oh-ma)

A cancerous growth in the pancreas that triggers hypoglycemia. The growth prevents glucose levels from being in check, thus reducing the body's blood sugar levels.

Interstitial Cell-Stimulating Hormone

Also known as luteinizing hormone. A hormone produced by gonadotropic cells around the anterior pituitary gland. For men, the hormone supports the production of testosterone. For women, the hormone influences the body's natural ovulation cycle.

Juvenile Onset Diabetes

A form of diabetes that develops among children. This is also called Type I diabetes. The condition may be hereditary, although it could also signal a significant concern in the pancreas or other glands responsible for managing blood sugar levels.

Laparoscopy (lap-ar-os-caw-pee)

A surgical procedure where a small tube is inserted into a small opening in the body. The procedure helps treat glands, although it may also be used when a gland has to be removed. The practice reduces the effort needed to enter the patient's body.

Leptin

A hormone that controls the person's appetite, thus managing how energy is stored and used.

Luteinizing Hormone

A hormone produced by the pituitary gland to manage how sex hormones are produced. The hormone influences the ovary in the female body and the testes in the male. The production of ova and sperm is directly influenced by the LH that is generated.

Melatonin (mel-ah-tone-in)

A pineal gland hormone that influences a person's natural sleeping pattern.

Melanocyte Stimulating Hormone

One of the various hormones produced by the hypothalamus and pituitary gland. The cells support the release of melanin and melanocytes. The development helps in the production of healthy skin and hair. Hormones generated within the hypothalamus may directly influence how sexual functions develop in the body.

NIDDM

Noninsulin-dependent diabetes mellitus. Also known as Type II diabetes or adult-onset diabetes. The body either becomes incapable of handling insulin or is unable to produce the correct insulin level. The insulin is unable to transfer the glucose into the cells for energy.

Norepinephrine (nor-eh-pin-ef-rin)

A neurotransmitter produced in the blood in response to stress. The compound elevates blood pressure levels and supports the body's functionality when stressful events take place.

Oxytocin (ox-ee-to-sin)

A hormone produced by the hypothalamus and released through the posterior pituitary gland. The hormone supports labor contractions in the birthing process and may also keep bleeding from developing following childbirth. The hormone may also help support abortive processes. The hormone may also continue to develop in the female body after pregnancy and may support the bonding aspect between the mother and child.

Pancreatitis (pan-cree-at-eye-tis)

Inflammation in the pancreas.

Parathyroid Hormone

Parathyroid hormone, or PTH, is produced by the parathyroid gland with the intention of supporting the development of a healthy bone structure. This includes allowing bone tissues to be resorbed in the body and eventually rebuilt to become firm and strong. The hormone may also be found in those who have experienced low blood calcium levels.

Parathyroidectomy (pear-ah-thy-roid-eck-toe-mee)

The removal of a parathyroid gland by surgery. This may involve multiple glands.

Pituitary Adenoma (ad-eh-noe-ma)

A benign growth in the pituitary gland.

Pituitary Gland (pit-oo-e-tear-ee)

A gland that links to the hypothalamus through the infundibulum, a small strand of tissue. The gland assists in supporting growth and metabolic functions by producing hormones that regulate physical activities in the body.

Polydipsia (pol-ee-dip-see-a)

An excessive thirst.

Polyphagia (pol-ee-fay-gee-a)

Excess hunger.

Prolactin

A pituitary hormone that enhances lactation in the female body. The hormone is also called PRL and may be noticed the most in women who are pregnant or nursing. The hormone can also influence breast development and may be found in men experiencing gynecomastia.

Progesterone (pro-jess-tur-own)

A sex hormone generated by the ovaries.

Prolactinoma (pro-lack-tin-oh-mah)

A tumor found in the pituitary gland that leads to excess production of prolactin. The tumor is usually benign.

Puberty

The time when the body is first capable of experiencing sexual reproduction.

SIADH

Syndrome of inappropriate diuretic sexually. A condition where the body experiences an excess amount of antidiuretic hormone. The condition may cause the body to retain more water than what it can handle. The water is not removed through the urination process, while the sodium content in the body might become excessive due to an imbalance of electrolytes.

Somatotrophs (soe-ma-toe-trofs)

Pituitary cells that create human growth hormone.

Steroids

Hormones generated in the body to help treat swelling and other athletic concerns. The hormones are often used to try to enhance the body's athletic performance. Steroids may be administered through various medications, although that is illegal.

Thyroxine (thigh-rocks-een)

Also called T4 - a hormone produced by the thyroid gland. This is an inactive hormone that is converted into triiodothyronine or T3 by the liver and kidneys.

Triiodothyronine (try-oh-doe-thy-roe-neen)

Also called T3 - a thyroid hormone that influences body temperature, metabolic rate, and heart rate.

Testosterone (tess-toss-ter-own)

A hormone produced by the testicles in men. The compound helps maintain the body's muscle mass and bone density. This may also influence a person's sexual drive. The hormone is found in men, although it may also be produced by a woman's ovaries in minimal amounts.

Thymosin (thigh-moe-sen)

A hormone produced by the thymus. The hormone generates T-cells needed to fight various diseases in the body.

Thyroid (thigh-roid)

An endocrine gland that regulates metabolic functions in the body. The gland has two lobes that are linked together by a small piece of tissue. The thyroid lobes are found on the sides of the trachea.

Thyroidectomy (th-eye-roid-eck-toe-mee)

A surgical procedure to remove the thyroid gland. This is conducted by the use of a laparoscope.

Thyroiditis (th-eye-roid-eye-tis)

Inflammation in the thyroid gland.

Thyroxine (thy-rox-een)

A hormone produced by the thyroid gland that regulates how the body consumes oxygen.

TSH

Thyroid-stimulating hormone. The hormone is produced in the pituitary gland and will stimulate the thyroid gland's functions. TSH assists in the production of T4 and T3 to support the metabolic functions of tissues throughout the body.

Vipoma (v-eye-poe-ma)

An endocrine tumor that produces vasoactive intestinal peptide. The compound will cause smooth muscles to relax and vasodilation. Diarrhea may be produced with an intense loss of body fluids, particularly water in the body.

Prefixes

acr	extremities
aden/o	gland
adren/o	adrenal gland
cortic/o	cortex or outside part of the body
crin/o	secretion

gluco	glucose
glyc/o	glucose or sugar
myx	muus
pancreat	pancreas
pituitary	pituitary
thalam	thalamus
thym	thymus gland
thry	thyroid gland

Chapter 4 – Eye and Ear Health

The following list of terms is health-related concerns regarding the eyes and ears. These terms may be used to identify how the eyes and ears are treated and how they may function. You may also notice some terms relating to conditions that are triggered over time or through some outside activities that a person may develop. These conditions may be treated by a specialist devoted to the eyes and ears.

Abducens Nerve (ahb-due-sins)

A cranial nerve near the pons. The nerve helps send motor fibers towards the lateral rectus muscles in the eye. The nerve influences how the eye moves horizontally.

Adnexa (ad-necks-ah)

The individual parts of an organ. The adnexa most often refers to the eyelids and how they cover the eyeball.

Alacrima (al-ah-crim-a)

Dry eye or a condition where the eyes are not getting the moisture they require.

Amaurosis (am-or-oh-sis)

Blindness triggered by a disease. The blindness might be partial or complete.

Amblyopia (am-blie-oh-pee-a)

A lack of vision due to the tissues in the eye not developing properly during puberty. The condition may also be called lazy eye due to the eye not being easily controlled.

Ametropia (am-ee-troe-pee-a)

An eye issue developed by improper refraction.

Anisocoria (an-es-oe-core-ee-a)

When the pupil sizes in the eyes are uneven.

Anterior Chamber

A spot in between the iris and cornea. The area is filled with fluid to hydrate the space.

Aphakia (af-ak-ee-ah)

When the eye's lens is missing. The condition may develop issues like farsightedness or hyperopia. A patient may be at an elevated risk of developing glaucoma or the detachment of the retina from the rest of the eye tissue.

Aqueous Humor

A fluid found within the eye. This is a clear fluid that helps hydrate the tissue and promotes proper movements in the tissue. The fluid is found in between the anterior and posterior chambers in the eye.

ARMD

Age-related macular degeneration. The macula, a central part of the retina, is impacted as fatty deposits develop under the tissue. This causes vision loss and blurriness. The condition is progressive and becomes more significant over time.

Astigmatism

A condition where the curve on the eye is faulty. The issue may be treated. Also listed on a report as Ast.

Audiology

A study of hearing including how impairments in hearing may develop.

Audiometry

A test to identify how well a person hears. The test is a series of various tones at different frequencies and intensities to identify how well the person can hear the sounds.

Aural

Relating to hearing.

Basilar Membrane (bas-il-ur)

A membrane found in the cochlea. The surface supports the hair cells located in the organ of Corti.

Biconcave (by-con-kave)

A concave found on both sides. The surface will curve inward like the inside part of the sphere. This is similar to what people notice in a lens.

Biconvex (by-con-vex)

The opposite of a biconcave, the biconvex occurs when a convex appears on both sides. The surface curves outward like the outside part of a sphere. The feature may also be noticed in a lens design.

Binaural (by-nor-ul)

Relating to both ears.

Binocular (byd-nock-u-lur)

Relating to both eyes.

Blepharitis (ble-far-eye-tis)

Inflammation that develops in the eyelids.

Blepharoplasty (ble-far-oh-plas-tee)

An eyelid lift. The eyelids are operated on to make the tissues look more attractive.

Blepharospasm (ble-far-oh-spa-zim)

Winking that develops in the eyelid due to the muscle in the region contracting without much control.

Blindness

When a person is unable to see. This may be a partial concern where a person can see things but not well, but it may also refer to a total loss of sight where the person cannot see at all. Further testing is required to gauge the intensity of the blindness that the person is experiencing.

Blinking

An event where the eyelids close and open. The condition occurs very quickly. Tests may help identify if the blinking is voluntary or not.

Cerumen (ser-u-min)

Also known as earwax - a series of secretions that are generated by sweat glands in the external ear canal.

Chalazion (chal-a-zee-on)

A bump located on the eyelid. The development that is produced due to an oil gland being blocked. The bump can be found around the end of the eyelash.

Choroid (koe-royd)

A layer located between the retina and sclera.

Choroiditis (kor-oid-eye-tis)

Inflammation in the choroid part of the eye.

Cochlea (coke-lee-ah)

The part of the inner ear that affects hearing. The section will help improve how a person can hear properly.

Cochlear Implant

A small implant that is provided to a patient who has hearing difficulties, particularly those who are deaf. The implant will provide a sense of sound to the person.

Color Blindness

A concern where a person is unable to distinguish colors. The blindness may be in various forms including cases where a person is unable to distinguish one specific color from another.

Conjunctiva (con-junk-tee-vah)

A mucous membrane on the posterior surface of the eyelids and the anterior surface of the eyeball. The compound covers the inside surface of the eyelids and allows proper hydration of the eyeballs.

Conjunctivitis (con-junk-tiv-eye-tis)

Also known as pink eye - an inflammation of the tissue along the white part of the eye. The tissue may be noticed as having a pink-like appearance, hence the name.

Cornea

A transparent part of the eye. This is the area that reflects light to provide the eyeball with improved sight in various light conditions.

Corneal Edema

Development of excess fluid in the cornea. The concern develops due to the epithelium not working accordingly. This includes a potential for visual acuity to decline.

Dacryoadenitis (dackro-a-den-eye-tis)

Inflammation in the lacrimal glands or the glands responsible for producing tears.

Dacryocystitis (dack-ro-sigh-stit-eye-tis)

Inflammation in the sac around the lacrimal gland.

Dark Adaptation

A change in how the pupil and retina may work. The change can be impacted by low light conditions. The eyes may become excessively sensitive to light.

Decibel

A measurement unit to identify the intensity of the sound. This includes the intensity of the electrical signal that produces sound. The measurement can be represented by the symbol dB and may refer to how well a person can hear sound.

Deafness

A basic measurement of how a person has lost the ability to hear. This is a condition that may involve either or both ears. Also, the deafness may be partial and will involve a portion of hearing being impacted. In other cases, the person may be completely deaf.

Diopter (dye-op-tur)

A measurement of how refractive a lens is.

Diplopia (dip-loe-pee-ah)

Double vision

Dry Eye Syndrome

A concern where the eyes are dry due to not producing enough tears. This may be a concern around the conjunctival and corneal parts of the eyes.

Ear

An organ that assists in hearing. The ear will collect vibrations from sounds and then convert those vibrations into nerve signals that will go through the tissue and eventually to the central nervous system.

Earache

General pain in the ear organ

Ectropion (eck-troe-pee-on)

An issue where the low eyelid drops past the eye. The eyelid may move outward, thus keeping the eye from being covered. This may also cause concerns where the eye moves outward.

EENT

A general term used to refer to the eye, ear, nose, and throat. This may refer to a specialist who deals with these aspects of the body.

Emmetropia

An eye that does not have any defects. In this case, rays will focus properly along the eye's retina. This is interpreted as a person having ideal vision and may be found in either or both eyes.

Entropion (en-troe-pee-on)

When the eyelid is rolled inward towards the eye.

Epiphora (ep-eep-or-ah)

The production of excess tears. This is due to the lacrimal duct being blocked.

Episclera (ep-is-klar-ah)

The tissues that link the sclera and conjunctiva.

Episcleritis (ep-is-klar-eye-tis)

Inflammation in the sclera. The issue may cause redness in the eye.

Esotropia (es-oh-troe-pee-ah)

When one or both eyes are turned inward.

Exotropia (ex-oh-troe-pee-ah)

When one or both eyes are turned outward.

Eyebrow

A bony structure that is over the eye socket. The surface protects the main part of the eye. The eyebrow may also refer to the hair that grows on the surface.

Eyelashes

A series of hairs that develop along the edges of the eyelids.

Floater

A string that appears to move along the eye. The floater may develop along the line of vision and may cloud one's vision on occasion.

Fluorescein Angiography (floor-es-sin an-ge-oh-gra-fee)

A test that identifies how well a retina and choroid are functioning. This involves the use of a dye and camera to identify how well blood flows into the retina and choroid. The dye is applied through a dropper.

Focus

An area where rays of light will link to one another after going through the lens.

Glare

A light that will impair one's vision. This may include the eyes being blinded due to the light being too intense.

Glaucoma (glau-koe-mah)

A condition where pressure levels in the eye increase. The concern may cause the optic nerve to be damaged.

Hearing Distance

The ability of a person to hear sound over a distance.

Hemianopia (hem-ee-an-oh-pee-ah)

When the eyes lose part of its field of vision on one side. The concern often develops due to damages to the brain, most often due to a stroke.

Heterophoria (het-er-oh-for-ee-ah)

When the eyes might not be parallel with one another. This may cause the eyes to focus on different things at one time.

Hippus (hip-us)

Regular dilation and constriction in the pupils. The changes occur at a rhythm and will continue to do so regardless of how the light changes.

Hordeolum (hor-de-oh-lum)

When a gland in the eyelid is blocked by a cyst. Inflammation may develop in this case.

Hyperopia (high-per-oh-pee-ah)

A person experiencing farsightedness. In this case, a person can see distant objects well, but closer items are not capable of coming in focus.

Hyphema (high-feem-ah)

Bleeding around the eye's anterior chamber.

Infectious Myringitis (my-ring-eye-tis)

An infection where the eardrums develop blisters. The condition can be infectious and transmitted to others, although it is more likely to be found in children than adults.

Iridectomy (ir-ed-ect-to-mee)

When a part of the iris is surgically removed. This occurs when the tissue develops an intense form of inflammation.

Iridoplegia (ir-ee-doh-plee-jah)

Paralysis of a muscle in the iris or dilator area that may keep the tissue from working properly.

Iris

A circular tissue behind the cornea. The membrane provides the eye with its visible color. The iris is also located outside the pupil.

Iritis (eye-reye-tis)

When the iris becomes inflamed.

Keratitis (care-aht-eye-tis)

Inflammation in the cornea.

Keratoconjunctivitis (care-ah-toe-con-junk-tev-eye-tis)

Inflammation in the cornea and conjunctiva.

Keratoconus (care-ah-toe-con-us)

A protrusion found in the middle part of the cornea, usually in a conical shape.

Labyrinth (lab-rin-the)

A series of ducts in the ear required for hearing and balance. The area is also called the inner ear.

Labyrinthectomy (lab-rin-theck-toe-mee)

An operation that treats Meniere's syndrome. The procedure will cause the balance organs to be removed so the brain will not receive signals from the inner ear. This may negatively influence the patient's hearing but would be required for controlling vertigo, tinnitus, and other related conditions.

Labyrinthitis (lab-rin-thy-tis)

Inflammation in the inner ear.

Lacrimation (lac-rim-ay-shun)

The process of crying and producing tears.

Laser Trabeculoplasty (tra-beck-ue-loe-plas-tee)

A common procedure for treating glaucoma. A laser will drain the aqueous fluid that may influence the condition. The effort also reduces the pressure levels in the eyes by easing the tissues.

Macula Lutea (mack-ue-lah lu-tee-ah)

A spot found in the retina. This is yellow and oval in appearance and does not have any retinal blood vessels with the exception of in the periphery area.

Macular (mack-u-lur)

Referring to the central retina.

Macular Degeneration

Destruction of the retina where the central visual field is impaired. The condition is caused by fatty deposits in the area. This may develop at any point in life, although it may also be an age-related condition.

Maculopathy (mack-ue-loe-path-ee)

A condition where the macula lutea is influenced negatively.

Malleus (mal-e-us)

Also known as the hammer. This is the largest bone found in the ear.

Mastoid (mas-toid)

A bone located behind the ear. This is a part of the temporal bone and supports the movement of blood through vessels. This includes the proper movement of blood through the ears to improve hearing.

Mastoidectomy (mas-toid-eck-toe-mee)

The surgical removal of the mastoid air cells in the skull behind the ear.

Mastoiditis (mas-toid-eye-sis)

Inflammation in the mastoid air cells. This may be caused by otitis media.

Meibomian Glands (may-boe-mee-in)

Small glands found along the inside surfaces of the eyelids.

Miosis (my-oh-sis)

When the pupils constrict more than necessary.

Miotics (my-ah-tix)

Drugs that cause the pupils to contract.

Mydriasis (my-dree-ah-sis)

A concern where the pupils become dilated too often or at the wrong times.

Myopia (my-oh-pee-ah)

Nearsightedness. This is when a person can see close items clearly but struggles to see far off items.

Myringitis (my-ring-eye-tis)

Inflammation in the eardrum.

Myringotomy (my-ring-oh-toe-mee)

A surgical procedure that relieves fluid pressure in the eye. An opening is made in the eardrum to reduce the pressure.

Nasolacrimal Duct (nay-soe-lack-ri-mul)

A duct that moves tears from the lacrimal gland over to the nose.

Nictation (nick-tay-shun)

A reflex known as blinking. The eyelids move up and down in moments. The process may be involuntary or intentional.

Night Blindness

A concern when a person is unable to see in dark conditions. This may also be called nyctalopia.

Nystagmus (nigh-stag-mus)

A concern where the eyes make consistent movements without control. The movements are noticed as the eyes move side to side.

Ocular Absorption

When the eye tissues begin to take in certain medications or other items.

Ocular Hypertension

When the intraocular pressure in the eyes is higher than usual. The concern may result in glaucoma.

Ocular Hypotension

When the intraocular pressure declines. The concern may lead to frequent inflammation of the tissue.

Oculomotor (ock-ue-loe-mo-ter)

Relating to eye movements.

Ophthalmia (op-thal-mee-ah)

Inflammation in the eye.

Ophthalmoplegia (op-thal-moe-ple-gee-ah)

Paralysis in one of the ocular muscles.

Ophthalmoscopy (op-thal-moe-sco-pee)

A review of the back part of the eye including the retina, choroid, and blood vessels. A dilating agent is required to expand the pupil to enhance the test. A light will also be used to identify how the area is functioning.

Optic Nerve

The second cranial nerve that allows visual data to go from the retina to the brain.

Optic Neuritis

A concern where the optic nerve develops inflammation.

Optic Tract

A nerve fiber that connects the optic nerve region to the lateral geniculate area. The tract helps supports the transmission of visual data to different regions with an emphasis on supporting the optic nerves.

Orbital Myositis

Inflammation around the eye's outside muscles. This may be noticed as swelling in the tissue.

Ossicle (oss-ick-ul)

A small bone found in the middle ear. The bone helps to move sounds in the air to the cochlea.

Otalgia (oat-al-gee-ah)

Pains in the ear.

Otitis (oht-eye-tis)

Inflammation in the ear. This may produce vertigo and other hearing issues or pains.

Otitis Media (me-de-ah)

An ear infection found in the middle ear or a spot located behind the eardrum.

Otomycosis (oh-toe-my-coe-sis)

A fungal infection that develops in the auditory canal. The condition appears mainly along the outside part of the ear.

Otopyorrhea (oh-toe-pie-or-hea)

A condition where pus comes out of the ear.

Otosclerosis (oh-toe-scl-er-oe-sis)

A condition where the tissues in the middle and inner ears are not functioning properly.

Otoscope

A tool used to analyze the inner ear. The unit is placed into the ear canal and will produce a light to help the doctor identify any concerns that might be found inside the ear.

Panuveitis (pan-oov-eye-tis)

Inflammation in the uvea tract. This includes inflammation in multiple parts of the tissue.

Papilledema (pap-il-ed-em-ah)

Swelling in the optic disk. The concern develops due to an increase in intracranial pressure.

Pupillary Distance

A measure of the distance between the pupils. This is a measurement in millimeters. The measurement is taken from the centers of the pupils. The analysis is done to determine how prescription eyewear is to be produced for a patient. The PD should be from 58 to 68 mm in length, although this may be closer to 62 mm for women or 64 mm for men.

Periorbital Edema (per-ee-or-bit-ul)

A concern where the tissues surrounding the eyes swell due to fluid buildup. The condition may also be called puffy eyes.

PERRLA

A measure stating that the pupils are equal and regular and can react to light and accommodation. The measure suggests that the eyes are healthy and little corrective procedures are required.

Photalgia (foe-tal-gee-ah)

Pains in the eyes that are caused by intense light exposure.

Photophobia (foe-toe-foe-bee-ah)

An unusual case of light sensitivity in the eyes.

Photoretinitis (foe-toe-ret-in-eye-tis)

An injury to the retina. This may be caused by the person looking directly into the sun without proper eye protection.

Presbycusis (press-by-cue-sis)

Hearing loss that develops mainly among those who get older.

Presbyopia (press-by-oh-pee-ah)

A condition where the eye lens does not change shape very well. The condition is associated with rigidity and may be more prominent among those who are older.

Proptosis (prop-toe-sis)

A condition where the eye bulges by a small amount.

Pseudophakia (sue-doe-fa-kee-ah)

When an intraocular lens appears after a cataract is surgically removed from the eye.

Ptosis (toe-sis)

A concern where the upper eyelid droops.

Pupil (pue-pul)

A small black spot in the iris. This is the area where light passes through. The pupil may constrict or dilate depending on the conditions or how the eye functions.

Radial Keratotomy (care-ah-toe-toe-me)

A surgical procedure that reduces the intensity of nearsightedness. The cornea is cut open and then reshaped. The procedure is typically conducted with laser technology and may be referred to as LASIK surgery.

Retina

A layer found on the inside part of the eye. The retina receives images that have been transmitted through the lens. The retina also includes the rods and cones, the two receptors needed for promoting accurate vision.

Retinitis (ret-in-eye-tis)

Inflammation in the retina.

Retinopexy (ret-in-oh-pecks-ee)

A surgical procedure used to control retinal detachment. The procedure is typically completed with a freezing material or laser to inject gas into the eye to help reattach the retina. A laser may also be used to seal the tissue.

Saccades (sack-aids)

A sudden shift in how well the eyes can focus on certain things. The concern may be noticed the most when a person is reading.

Saccule (sack-yul)

A membrane sac that is found inside the vestibule along the inner ear. The saccule contains a fluid that responds to sound vibrations and changes in gravity. The tissue also gives the brain information about the head's position for proper balance control.

Sclera (sc-ler-ah)

A white part on the outside area of the eyeball. The sclera covers much of the eye with the exception of the cornea.

Scleritis (sc-ler-eye-tis)

An inflammation that develops in the sclera. The condition is very significant and could potentially cause blindness.

Scotoma (skoe-toe-mah)

An area of declined vision within the visual field.

Scotopic (scoe-toe-pick)

How the eye can conform to low light conditions. This includes looking at how well the eye works in some difficult conditions where the light is not present.

Semicircular Canals

A series of canals that come out from the labyrinth. These are also known as the anterior, posterior, and lateral canals. These are positioned at right angles to one another and will support the brain's ability to handle a sense of balance.

Sensorineural Hearing Loss

The loss that develops due to hearing issues in the inner ear.

Snow Blindness

A condition where the eyes are damaged due to exposure to ultraviolet rays without protection. The condition is also called photokeratitis. The issue might cause intense pains in the eyes.

Stapedectomy (stape-ect-toe-mee)

Surgical procedure on a stape in the ear.

Stape

An ossicle found in the middle ear. A person has three of these ossicles. The stape transmits sound vibrations from the outside of the ear to the inner ear.

Strabismus (stra-bis-mus)

A condition where a person develops crossed eyes.

Stye (sty)

A bacterial inflammation that develops along with the gland on the end of an eyelash that is attached to the skin of the eyelid.

Tarsorrhaphy (tar-sore-ha-fee)

When a part of the upper and lower eyelids are connected to each other. The condition develops to close the eye, sometimes partially but completely in more cases.

Tears

A term for the fluids that are produced by the lacrimal glands. The fluids are triggered to keep the cornea and conjunctiva hydrated. A lack of tears may result in dry eye conditions, thus triggering intense pain.

Tectorial Membrane (teck-tore-ee-ul)

A membrane in the cochlea that is alongside the basilar membrane.

Tinnitus (tin-eye-tus)

The sound that develops in the head even when there is no outside sound in the area. This is a concern also known as ringing in the ears due to the consistent sound.

Tonometry

A test that identifies the fluid pressure or intraocular pressure inside the eye. The test involves a gust of air applied on the eye to identify the pressure level.

Trachoma (track-oh-mah)

An infection that regularly develops in the conjunctiva and cornea. The condition may be caused by a bacterial infection.

Trichiasis (trick-ee-ah-sis)

A growth of ingrown hair around a part of the face. The condition develops mostly along the eyelashes. Ingrown hair can result in pain in the tissue and extensive irritation.

Tympanic Cavity (tim-pan-ick)

A small cavity that is found over the middle ear bones. The cavity is where the ossicles are located to transfer sound vibrations to other parts of the ear and eventually to the brain.

Tympanic Membrane (tim-pan-ick)

A small membrane that divides the outside ear canal from the tympanic cavity.

Tympanocentesis (tim-pan-oh-sen-tee-sis)

A process where the tympanic membrane is punctured and fluid is cleared from the middle ear. This is often a needle aspiration process to relieve pressure in the area and possibly to clear an infection.

Tympanometry (tim-pan-owe-met-tree)

A test of the middle ear to determine how well the eardrum functions. The ear canal is treated with varying amounts of air pressure to identify how well the bones in the region can conduct sounds and respond.

Uvea (oo-vee-ah)

A pigmented part of the eye. The layer appears beneath the cornea and sclera. The iris, choroid, and ciliary body are all parts of the uvea.

Uveal (oo-ve-al)

Relating to the uvea.

Uveitis (oo-vee-eye-tis)

Inflammation in the uvea.

Visual Acuity

A measure of how sharp a person's vision is. The measurement indicates a person's ability to identify numbers at a distance. The measure is based on a certain standard for normality. A Snellen chart that lists a series of letters and numbers of varying sizes may be used. A person who has 20/20 vision according to the visual acuity test is said to have normal vision.

Vertigo (vur-tig-oh)

A condition where a person feels dizzy and disoriented. This may be due to impairments in the ear that affects the person's sense of balance. The issue provides a false sense of moving or spinning even when the body is still. This may be triggered by a sudden change in one's head position or when someone experiences fatigue. Vertigo may be a sign of a possible tumor, although not all people who experience vertigo have a tumor.

Vf

A reference to one's field of vision. This is a measurement of how well a person is able to see things at many angles.

Vitrectomy (vit-rek-toe-mee)

A surgical procedure where the vitreous body in the eye is removed. The procedure allows the surgeon to have better access to the retina. The treatment is performed to repair a retinal detachment or when scar tissue has to be removed.

Vitreous Body (vit-ree-us)

A gelatinous compound found in the cavity behind the eye lens and in front of the retina. The surface has a transparent appearance.

Xerophthalmia (ze-roe-thal-mee-ah)

A condition where dry eyes develop. The issue may be significant and can be caused by the tear glands not operating normally.

Prefixes

acou   relating to hearing

anbly/o   dull or dim

audi/o	relating to hearing
aur/o	ear
blephar/o	eyelid
cerumen/o	earwax
cochle/o	cochlea
conjunctiv/o	conjunctiva
cor	pupil
corne	cornea
dacry/o	tears and tear production
hygr/o	moisture and how well the eye handles the compound
irid/o	iris
kerat/o	cornea; this may also refer to a hard surface
labyrinth/o	inner ear
lacrim	tears
logad	white parts of the eyes
macul	spot
myring	eardrum
ocul/o	relating to the eye
ophry/o	eyebrow
ophthalm/o	eye
opt/o	eye or vision-related
ot/o	ear or hearing
palperbr/o	eyelid
phac	relating to the lens
phak	relating to the lens

phot/o	light
pupill/o	pupil
retin/o	retina
scler/o	white part of the eye
scot/o	dark conditions or lack of vision
son/o	sound
staped/o	stapes, a bone in the middle ear
trop/o	turn
tympan/o	eardrum
uve	uvea
vitre	vitreous body

Chapter 5 – Integumentary System

The integumentary system is a part of the body that includes the skin and other features that will protect the body from many external threats. The system includes the hair and nails and other features that appear on the external part of the body. This chapter refers to many of the conditions that may develop in the integumentary system.

Acne (ack-knee)

Inflammation in the sebaceous glands and hair follicles. The issue develops as oil is backed up in parts of the tissues. This may cause painful bumps to develop with some sore spots appearing. Noticeable oil buildup may also appear; these may leak depending on the amount of pressure that is caused. The condition is likely to develop in puberty, although it could occur at any time due to various concerns surrounding the body's hormonal responses and dietary concerns that may develop.

Acne Conglobata (con-gloe-bah-tah)

Severe acne. Also called cystic acne. The acne is chronic and will produce intense cysts that go deep into the skin. The condition can be scarring and will cause disfigurement of the skin.

Acne Keloid (kel-oyd)

A disorder where a secondary infection will develop in scarring. The pustules that form will be deep in intensity and can occur on the scalp and rear part of the neck. The condition is likely to develop in young black men more than others.

Acrodermatitis (ack-roe-der-maht-eye-tis)

Inflammation in the skin in the hands and feet. This may be caused by a parasite. Acrodermatitis is a possible sign of Lyme disease. Red and purple blisters may start to form around the body. Children under the age of 15 years are at a higher risk of developing the condition.

Actinic Keratosis (ack-tin-ick ker-a-toe-sis)

A pre-cancerous patch of skin. The scaly or thick skin will develop due to the body being exposed to the sun's rays for lengthy periods of time.

Actinomycosis (ack-tin-oh-my-coe-sis)

A bacterial disease that is caused by the Actinomyces species. This is an infection that can produce abscesses in the body. These will produce pus that may discharge from the body at random. The condition is likely to be found in the abdomen, although it may also occur on the thorax and jaw.

Adenocarcinoma (ey-den-oh-car-sin-oh-mah)

Cancer that starts in the body's glands and will transfer to other parts of the body. The glands will secrete many fluids into tissues that line the body's organs. The tumor-associated with cancer will have a glandular appearance.

Albinism (al-bin-ism)

A genetic condition where a person's skin, hair, or eyes do not have any or very little color.

Algid (al-gid)

Cold skin associated with malaria.

Aloe (al-oe)

A juice that comes from the aloe plant leaf. The juice may be dried and prepared in an ointment. The compound will help treat various burns and forms of irritation. Aloe may also be a hydrating agent that helps the body to retain its natural store of moisture.

Alopecia (al-oe-pee-sha)

A condition where the immune system attacks the scalp's hair follicles. The condition causes a person to lose their hair. The existing hair may also become weak and brittle and may not grow back the way it should normally.

Anetoderma (an-et-oh-dur-mah)

A benign form of dermatosis that is triggered by a loss of dermal elastic tissue. The condition will produce small flaccid skin spots. The condition can make it harder for the body to function properly.

Angioedema (an-ge-oh-ed-eem-ah)

A form of swelling that develops in the dermis or subcutaneous tissues. The condition may develop in the face, lips, tongue, or larynx.

Angiokeratoma (an-ge-oh-ker-a toe-mah)

A benign lesion of capillaries. The condition results in several red and blue marks on the skin. The condition may appear on the legs and feel.

Angioma (an-gee-oh-ma)

A benign tumor that includes blood vessels and lymph nodes. The vessels can cause some redness and other spots on the skin and may trigger pains depending on how intense the tumor is. Although the tumor is non-threatening in most cases, there are times when an angioma may become malignant. Some angiomas may also be likely to develop with age, although age-related spots may be a natural concern for most to experience.

Angiomyoma (an-gee-oh-my-oh-ma)

A benign smooth muscle tumor. The condition develops in the vessel walls in the body. This can develop in many areas around the body and can influence the lower limbs in females and upper limbs in males.

Antiperspirant (an-tee-per-spir-int)

A compound that is applied topically to prevent or reduce sweating. Deodorant is the most noteworthy type of antiperspirant to use.

Antipruritic (an-ty-pru-rit-ick)

An agent that controls itching. This is a topical compound in most cases.

Apocrine Glands (ap-i-creen)

Sweat glands that can be found in the hairiest areas of the body.

Argyria (ar-guy-re-ah)

A condition that develops due to excess exposure to silver dust or the silver element. The condition will cause the skin to develop a purple or purple-grey tint. Those who use colloidal silver for treatments, particularly when ingesting the compound, may develop the condition. The internal organs may also develop the same pigmentation and could be at risk of harm depending on how intense the condition is.

Barrier Cream

A cream that will be applied to the skin to prevent the tissue from allergens and other threats.

Basal Cell Carcinoma (bay-sul)

A malignant form of skin cancer. Cancer develops on parts of the skin that are frequently exposed to the sun. The condition may be noticed by a rising mark that features a visible central ulcer. A rolled border that forms a circular appearance may develop due to cancer. A white lump may also develop in some cases. A surgical procedure may be required to remove the cancer growth. The risk of metastasis is minimal in this case.

Biopsy (by-op-see)

A procedure a doctor will perform to surgically remove tissue from the skin. The process allows some of the skin to be examined to identify any possible growths or other abnormalities. A complete exam can find the cause of a disease or how extensive the disease might have become. May be abbreviated in a report as Bx.

Birthmark

A benign spot that appears at birth. The spot appears due to blood vessels growing more than needed. Smooth muscle, fat, or fibroblasts may also cause some birthmarks to appear. The condition may happen during the first month of one's life. Some birthmarks may disappear or become less noticeable over time.

Blackhead

A small bit of fatty material that develops in the sebaceous gland in the skin. A blackhead may be found in a clogged hair follicle. The surface will have a black look to it. This is a form of acne that may be hard and rough while producing some soreness. The blackhead may also develop on the face, although it could appear on the back of the upper chest.

Blister

A growth of watery fluid that builds up within or under the epidermis. The blister may become sore and could open if too much pressure is applied in the area. An appropriate sterile dressing should be applied over the blister in the event the tissue bursts open and starts to leak. This is to prevent a possible infection from developing.

Boil

A tender spot on the skin that is associated with acne. The area may develop inflammation and can also include pus, which may leak depending on the pressure caused.

Bruise

A type of contusion that appears on the skin due to a form of trauma. This may occur from excess pressure on the body or from a cut. The injury will cause a series of capillaries under the skin to burst. This can cause temporary discoloration and soreness in the area. It may take a few days or weeks to recover from the bruise depending on the severity.

Bulla (bue-lah)

A blister that is at least 5 millimeters in diameter. The blister includes fluid, usually pus.

Burn

An injury that is produced due to outside material. A burn can be triggered by extreme heat or cold conditions, exposure to chemicals, electricity, radiation, or ultraviolet light. A first-degree burn would involve the top part of the skin, while a second-degree burn will go deeper. A third-degree burn can cut into the fatty tissues in the skin and may cause some of the internal parts of the skin to be exposed.

Calamine (kal-ah-mine)

A medicated lotion compound. The material is applied to the skin to dry out areas that may be irritated. This may also treat itchiness caused by poison plant exposure, insect bites, and other skin conditions.

Capillary Hemangioma (he-man-gee-oh-mah)

Also known as a strawberry birthmark. The benign tumor develops due to a series of capillaries growing more than normal. This may appear during the first few months of the child's life and could eventually disappear after 12 to 15 months of age. However, some do not disappear.

Carbuncle (kar-bun-cull)

A red series of pus-filled bumps and boils. The tissues link to an infection that will develop under the skin. Pus may be found on the skin in the neck, although the shoulders and thighs may also develop some concerns. The pus pocket will eventually rupture and drain.

Cellulitis (cell-ue-l-eye-tis)

A bacterial skin infection. This may develop as a red and swollen area that will feel hot and tender when you touch it. The redness can spread fast and result in intense pain. The bacteria will enter the skin and may spread to cover many areas. This can go into the dermis in the most significant cases.

Chafing (chay-fing)

Irritation to the skin that is triggered by a surface rubbing on the area. The concern develops mainly due to skin and clothing.

Chancre (kan-cur)

A syphilis sore. The sore appears around the site where the infection started. This may result in an ulcer, although the condition should be painless.

Chancroid (kan-croid)

A bacterial disease that is transmitted through sexual contact. This is also be called a venereal ulcer. The disease causes open sores to develop in the genital area. Men and women alike can be affected.

Chapping

A process where the skin starts to become dry and cracked. Redness may develop in some cases. A lack of moisture or the sudden evaporation of that moisture will influence the problem. Chapping frequently develops in the hands.

Chigger (chig-gur)

Also known as a berry bug. The chigger is a red-tinted arachnid that can transfer a skin rash. The arachnid will often drain blood from the patient and can cause a sore or intense irritation to develop in the impacted area.

Chloasma (cloe-as-mah)

A condition where brown patches start to develop on the face. The patches are benign and may be triggered by hormonal changes or from excess sun exposure. Pregnant women are more likely to experience such patches.

Cicatrix (sic-ah-trick)

A scar that appears on the skin after a wound heals. The scar develops due to the skin cells not functioning or dividing normally in the area of the injury.

Comedo (com-ed-oh)

Another word for a blackhead or clogged hair follicle. This is one of the most common acne-related concerns that a person may experience.

Complexion

The general appearance of one's facial skin. The complexion is based on the color and texture of the person's facial skin.

Contusion (con-tue-shin)

An injury triggered by a blow to the body that will not break the skin. This is also known as a bruise. The injury will develop and the area will swell and cause pain. The area may also have temporary discoloration.

Dander (dan-dur)

A material that the body sheds. The body will develop dander mainly along the scalp. The shedding will cause dry scales to develop.

Dandruff (dan-druf)

Shedding of scaly and dry skin cells from the scalp. This may be noticed through white flakes that may appear on the skin near the head. The flakes may also stay in the hair at times.

Debridement (de-bride-mint)

The removal of damaged tissue from a wound. Debridement may include the use of enzymes or the use of a surgical tool depending on the condition.

DEET

Diethyltoluamide. This is an oily compound that works as an insect repellent. The material may be applied on many surfaces on the body or on one's clothes to prevent insects from attacking the body and causing irritation.

Deodorant

A prominent type of antiperspirant. The compound will prevent odors and may also mask those odors.

Dermatitis (dur-mat-eye-tis)

Inflammation in the skin. An allergic reaction, drug use, or an infection of something may be a factor. A red and itchy rash may develop. This can also be called eczema. The condition can be chronic in some cases depending on how the body responds to certain treatments.

Dermis (dur-miss)

A layer of connective tissue that appears under the epidermis. The dermis includes hair follicles and nerves as well as various lymphatic vessels.

Desmosome (des-moe-some)

A structure in the body that includes two adjacent cells that connect to each other. The desmosome will connect from a protein plaque in the cell. The membranes are connected by filaments.

Diaper Rash

A concern that may develop in babies and infants. This is a form of dermatitis that appears on the thighs and buttocks. This is due to the baby's contact with urine or fecal matter.

Diaphoresis (dye-ah-four-ee-sis)

Sweating. The amount of sweating, in this case, may be intense. Diaphoresis may develop due to a side effect of a drug or another underlying condition.

Dysplasic Nevus (dis-plas-tick nev-us)

An unusual-looking mole. This may have an irregular shape and no defined border. The color of the mole may also vary in intensity. These moles are usually benign, but they may also be signs that a person could potentially develop melanoma in that area or on another area of the body.

Ecchymosis (eck-e-moe-sis)

Discoloration of the skin. The condition occurs due to bruising. The skin will bleed in its deepest layers. The bleeding should have a diameter of at least 1 centimeter for it to be considered an ecchymosis.

Eccrine Gland (eck-rin)

Sweat glands. These glands may be found in various parts of the skin, particularly in the soles and palms. Some of these glands may also be found on the head. The glands produce sweat that appears directly on the skin.

Eczema (ek-zima)

Inflammation in the skin that causes irritation and redness. Eczema may be triggered by hormonal changes and exposure to some dirt compounds. The intensity of the condition will vary.

Electrolysis (e-leck-trol-eh-sis)

A process for hair removal. An electric current is applied to the unwanted hair follicle. The follicle will shrink over time as multiple treatments are performed. The process works best for permanent hair removal and can be done on many parts of the skin. Some redness may develop on the treated area depending on the intensity.

Epidermis (ep-eh-dur-miss)

The surface part of the skin. This is an outside layer that is the primary source of protection for the body to prevent possible damages or threats to the skin.

Epilation (ep-il-a-shun)

The removal of hair by the root. An epilator is used to gather the hair and remove it from the follicle. The process removes the hair and keeps the area smooth. It may take a few weeks for the hair to grow back, although the quality of the hair will not change as it returns. Regular epilation treatment processes are needed at various times to keep the hair removed.

Epithelium (ep-eh-the-lee-um)

The cells that line hollow organs and glands. These cells also produce the outside part of the body.

Erysipelas (er-e-sip-el-ahs)

A skin infection. The bacterial infection will develop due to the Streptococcus bacteria getting on a scratch or other space. The condition can cause redness and some acute pains and chills. Antibiotic treatments are required to keep the condition under control.

Erythema (air-e-thee-mah)

A form of skin inflammation. The condition develops in the fatty parts of the skin. The capillaries in the area may become congested and cause harm depending on the intensity.

Erythrasma (air-e-thra-ss-mah)

An intense type of bacterial infection that can develop along the skin's folds. The condition is more likely to develop in warm and humid climates.

Erythroderma (air-ee-throw-dur-mah)

Reddening of the skin. The skin develops inflammation. The condition may spread over the entire body in some cases. The skin will exfoliate or start to peel off, thus causing exfoliative dermatitis to develop.

Eschar (ess-char)

A dead tissue piece that is shed from the skin after a burn or another infection. The condition develops mainly due to extreme fatigue or stress in the skin. The eschar is also referred to as a scab.

Exanthem (ex-an-them)

A rash that occurs with a fever, malaise, and a headache.

Exanthema (ex-an-theme-ah)

An eruption that develops on the skin. This is a sign of a disease.

Excoriation (ex-cor-ee-ay-shun)

A mental illness relating to obsessive-compulsive disorder or OCD. The condition causes a person to constantly pick at the skin. This may cause lesions and other disfiguring results. The issue occurs due to the patient being irritated or concerned over how the skin forms.

Exfoliation (ex-foal-e-a-shun)

A process where a layer of skin is removed. The procedure removes old skin cells that may have developed. Chemical agents or scrubs can be used in the exfoliation process, although the intensity of the results will vary based on the condition of the skin.

Exfoliative Dermatitis

Significant scaling along the skin. The condition can cause itching and redness. Hair loss may develop due to the top parts of the skin being shed quickly.

Flush

A blushing effect. The reddening develops in the facial tissues.

Follicle (fall-ick-ul)

A secretory cavity. This may be a sac or gland. The area is where hair roots are formed.

Folliculitis (fall-ee-cul-eye-tis)

An infection in the hair follicle.

Furuncles (fur-un-cls)

A boil that can develop in a hair follicle. The boil may be caused by a bacterial or fungal infection.

Granuloma (gran-u-loe-ma)

A tissue that is produced due to an infection or inflammation. This may be caused by a foreign substance that develops within the body. The immune system will attempt to clear harmful substances, but it will not remove the materials from the body. Foreign bodies may influence these cells.

Hair Follicle

A follicle that will support the production of hair. This is located in the epidermis and is where the hair shaft grows. The shaft allows the hair to grow as the sebaceous glands are open. A cellular inner and outer root sheath is produced in the process. The sheath comes from the epidermis. This may also include a fibrous sheath that is from the dermis.

Halitosis (hal-i-toe-sis)

Breath odor that develops due to improper oral hygiene. Particles of food may be left in the mouth that will produce sulfur materials when they break down, thus producing the unpleasant odor. Halitosis may be controlled by keeping the mouth hydrated to keep mouth odor from developing. Regular brushing and flossing are also needed to keep the mouth healthy and to prevent halitosis.

Hematoma (hee-mah-toe-mah)

A collection of blood outside of blood vessels that develops due to an injury to the wall of a blood vessel. This is also known as a bruise.

Hidrocystoma (high-dro-sis-toe-mah)

A sweat gland cyst. The adenoma or cyst is not a tumor, but it will cause the production of excess sweat in some cases.

Hidrosis (high-droe-sis)

The body's natural production of sweat.

Hidrotic (high-drot-ick)

Relating to sweating. This may also refer to something that causes sweating.

Hirsutism (her-suit-izm)

When a woman develops excess hair growth. This includes added hair around the legs, arms, and face. The hair growth occurs when a woman experiences a hormonal imbalance.

Hyalin (high-al-in)

A clear material produced in the body as a result of connective tissues dying. The material may stay on the skin and cause an uncomfortable glare depending on the intensity or spread.

Hyperhidrosis (high-pur-hy-droe-sis)

Excess sweating. The issue develops along the underarms as axillary hyperhidrosis or on the soles of the feet as palmoplantar hyperhidrosis. A prescription-grade antiperspirant may be required to take care of the condition.

Hyperpigmentation (high-pur-pig-men-tay-shun)

A condition where parts of the skin may become darker in tone than other parts of the skin. This may be due to the excess production of melanin. The melanin will produce a darker skin color at random places. The issue is not permanent, although it may take a few months for the issue to be treated properly.

Hypertrichosis (high-pur-trick-oh-sis)

Hair growth that develops in various locations. This includes growth around areas like the armpit and other places. The condition may occur around all parts of the body, but it can also develop smaller patches around many parts of the body.

Hypohydrosis (high-poe-hid-roe-sis)

A disorder where a person does not experience much sweating. The condition may cause heat stroke and hyperthermia in some cases due to the body not recognizing when the body is experiencing heat. The lack of sweat may also trigger problems relating to how well the body can stay hydrated.

Hypotrichosis (high-poe-try-ko-sis)

A condition where a person does not have enough hair on their body. This includes a lack of hair on the head. The condition is congenital and can be noticed mostly in the lack of hair in the eyebrows.

Ichthyosis (ick-ey-toe-sis)

A series of skin disorders that are noted by dry or thick skin.

Impetigo (im-pet-eye-goe)

Also known as school sores. The condition develops in children and appears as red sores around the face. The sores may burst and develop a series of crusted surfaces. The infection is contagious and can cause ruptures in the area. These sores may also ooze for a few days. Antibiotics can help the infection clear up.

Intertrigo (in-tur-tree-goe)

Inflammation produced in the warm and moist parts of the body including areas around the groin and between skin folds or under the breasts. This is a form of dermatitis that will develop in areas where skin surfaces are in a fold. People who experience intense moisture or friction in these tissues may experience these concerns.

Intraductal Papilloma (in-tra-duck-tul pap-il-oh-mah)

Benign tumors in the breast ducts.

Iodine (eye-oh-dine)

A nonmetallic element. The compound is used as a topical solution to prevent infections.

Keloid (kel-oid)

A growth of scar tissue around a wound. The tissue may inhibit the functionality of the impacted area.

Keratosis (care-ah-toe-sis)

A growth of skin that may feel horny and hollow. A wart or a callus may be interpreted as a keratosis.

Koilonychia (coil-on-ee-chee-ah)

A disease that develops in the fingernails. The nails will become thin and develop concave shapes.

Labial (lay-bee-ul)

Relating to the lip.

Lentigo (len-tee-go)

A pigmented spot on the skin. This is a small and flat surface.

Lichen (ly-kin)

A common skin disease that has small bumps or pimples occurring close together. The lesions are very small. The lichen may be a sign of a rash, although the bumps should not be interpreted as a sign of anything potentially malignant. Contacting and scratching the area may cause it to spread to other parts of the skin.

Liniments (lin-eh-mints)

Liquids that produce heat. The liquid is applied to the skin and may help relieve pains or irritation. Most liniments are made with an oil compound, although the construction of each liniment will vary based on what a patient may require.

Lipedema (lip-ed-eem-ah)

A condition where fatty tissues develop on the legs. The symmetric enlargement develops as fat deposits beneath the skin. The condition occurs mainly in women.

Lipoma (lip-oe-mah)

Benign growth of fatty cells. The cells develop in the body's tissues. These are more likely to appear in areas where a person has experienced trauma in the past.

Lupus (loop-us)

An inflammatory condition that does not have any cures, although treatments may help reduce the risk of flare-ups. The inflammation occurs when the immune system attacks its own tissues. This may cause fatigue, joint pain, and a butterfly rash. The condition may develop in the joints, skin, or various organs. The condition may be life-threatening depending on how it impacts certain organs in the body.

Macule (mack-yul)

A change in the color of something. The change is a spot becoming darker on the skin. The macule is flat and about 5 to 10 mm in diameter. The macule will be circular in most cases, although many small macules may combine with one another to create a larger macule.

Malignant Melanoma (mel-ah-noe-ma)

A dangerous type of skin cancer that involves a series of neoplasms that develop around the body. This may be a new growth or a change in a mole on the body. The melanoma may have a black or brown tone, although a white accent may appear in some malignant melanomas. The skin cancer will have an unusual shape. Treatment is required as soon as possible to prevent the melanoma from spreading.

Melanin (mel-ah-nin)

A natural pigment in the body that turns skin to a dark tone. The pigment is naturally dark brown or black and produces a person's dark skin tone. The pigment may also trigger tanning activities in the skin when the tissue is exposed to sunlight long enough.

Melanosis (mel-ah-noe-sis)

A condition where melanin production becomes too excessive. The added production causes the skin to become dark in various areas. The issue may develop without any prior inflammatory diseases.

Micrococcus (my-crow-cock-cus)

A bacteria with cells up to 3 micrometers in diameter.

Mite (might)

A small spider-like insect. The insect may be a parasite on human skin. The insect will trigger an intense irritation in the skin. Some mites may have transparent bodies and would be difficult for some people to notice.

Necrobiotic Disorder (neck-roe-by-ot-ic)

A disorder that involves collagen in the dermis being destroyed. This may be due to some collagen bundles swelling or deteriorating.

Necrotizing Fasciitis (neck-roe-ty-zing fas-ee-eye-tis)

A bacterial infection known as flesh-eating disease. The impact to soft tissue will develop when group A Streptococcus bacteria, or the flesh-eating bacteria, enters the body. The issue may develop within a break in the skin and can be dangerous to those who have weakened immune systems. The condition can include blisters, fatigue, and pain in the tissue while skin cells are killed off. The issue may spread fast along the body and can be deadly. Intravenous antibiotics are required besides the possible surgical removal of the dead tissue from the impacted area.

Neurodermatitis (new-roe-der-mat-eye-tis)

A condition loosely related to eczema. The condition develops as an itchy patch of skin that becomes worse when the patient scratches. The cycle of itching and scratching causes the tissue to become thick and to develop a leathery feel. This may develop in various areas, particularly around the anal area.

Nevus (nee-vuss)

A skin issue that is noticeable at birth. This may be a birthmark or mole. The nevus may develop due to issues surrounding the blood capillaries or the production of excess pigmented cells around certain parts of the skin tissue.

Ochronosis (ok-roe-no-sis)

Discoloration of body tissues. The condition develops into a metabolic disorder in the body. The tissues may not be negatively impacted, although the intensity of the condition may also be a factor that could influence what happens in the body.

Onychocryptosis (on-ee-ko-crip-toe-sis)

An ingrown toenail. The nail develops a fold that moves inward towards the nail bed. The nail plate may also develop unusual embedding in the nail groove causing serious discomfort in the patient's toenail area. This may be noted by redness along the corner of the toe. Those who engage in regular running activities may experience this condition. People who have diabetes will be at a higher risk of complications due to the ingrown toenail. Antibiotics are needed, although the toenail might have to be removed altogether.

Onychomycosis (on-ee-ko-my-coe-sis)

A nail fungus. The tinea unguium fungus will infect the nail. This may trigger the nail to become thick and could involve the nail being separated from the nail bed. The nail can also develop a white or yellow discoloration and a ragged appearance. A slight odor may also be triggered. Oral antifungal drugs are needed to treat the condition, although the nail itself might also have to be removed depending on the intensity of the issue.

Pallor (pal-or)

A pale appearance. This is a white look to the skin. The appearance may suggest that someone is unhealthy.

Panniculitis (pan-eh-cue-l-eye-tis)

Inflammation in the adipose tissue, particularly of the skin. The condition may be characterized by red nodules that develop all around. The skin will not have any raised bumps. Weight loss and fatigue may also be concerns.

Papilloma (pap-il-oh-mah)

A benign tumor in the skin or in a mucous membrane. The growth appears on the epidermis and may have a wart-like appearance. The condition may also be intraductal as it forms in the breast tissue, although this is not a sign of breast cancer or a suggestion that a woman would be at an elevated risk of cancer.

Papule (pap-ule)

A raised lesion on the body. The lesion is an effect of a skin condition and will have a significant border defining its shape. The lesion is less than 1 centimeter in diameter.

Paronychia (pear-on-e-chee-ah)

An infection in the skin near a nail. The infection may develop in the area under the nail and can include an intense and bright red spot with a raised area. This may be acute or sudden, or it could be a chronic condition that appears gradually and may occur even after it is initially treated. Antibiotics are needed to treat the condition. The pus inside the area may also have to be drained.

Pediculosis (ped-e-cue-loe-sis)

An infestation of lice. The condition may develop on any part of the body that has hair, although it is often associated with the head and the pubic area. The eggs or larvae of the lice insect may develop in the area and will consume the patient's blood around the skin. The issue will cause intense itching. The infestation is easily transmitted. Proper washing and cleaning are needed to treat an infestation, although the hair might have to be shaved off in the impacted area to potentially reduce the threats involved.

Pemphigus (pemph-eye-gus)

An autoimmune disorder. The immune system will attack healthy cells around the skin triggering blisters and sores. The condition is not contagious, although it is uncertain as to what causes it. Pemphigus is considered to be rare.

Perleche (pur-lay-chuh)

A crack that appears at the corners of the mouth. The crack may develop due to dryness or from a lack of zinc or other nutrients. Sores may develop and can cause a burning sensation. Antifungal treatments are required on the impacted areas. It is also called angular cheilitis.

Petechiae (pet-eek-ee-ay)

A series of patches that develop on a mucous membrane. These patches are red and small in size and may be paired with one another in one of many shapes. The patches develop due to bleeding under the skin. The patches can be produced around the extremities.

Piloerection (py-loe-ee-rec-shun)

When the hairs on the skin become erect. The hairs will stand up on the skin while a few raised bumps may also appear along those hairs. This can be due to exposure to cold temperatures, a shock, or another sudden event. The event may help keep the body warm by responding to the sudden change in the temperature in the skin.

Pilonidal Sinus (pieee-lon-ee-dul)

A cyst or sinus with hair. The tunnel will develop fluid and is likely to develop around the buttocks, specifically in the cleft area at the middle central part of the buttocks. The cyst may become infected if not treated properly. The skin may also become red.

Pinta (pin-tah)

A bacterial skin disease that is more likely to be found in tropical parts of the Americas. A papule forms at the beginning and is then followed by an eruption in the area. The pigment in the tissue may also be lost. The condition may be confused with syphilis.

Pityriasis (pit-ee-ray-sis)

A skin disease that is the production of fine scales along the body.

Porokeratosis (pour-oh-kar-ah-toe-sis)

A keratinization disorder. A series of atrophic patches will develop at one part of the body. The patches will appear round and small and may include raised borders. The condition is benign, although it is an issue that may trigger the development of skin cancer within the influenced area.

Poroma (pour-oh-mah)

A neoplasm of cells that forms in the openings of sweat glands.

Pressure Ulcer

An ulcer that develops in the skin over a bony tissue. The ulcer develops due to a lack of blood moving through and from excess pressure produced by compression. The condition is also known as bedsores. People who require extensive bedrest and wheelchair use are at elevated risk due to the added compression that may develop on parts of the body.

Prurigo (pru-ree-go)

Inflammation in the skin. The development occurs due to papules consistently erupting. The papules may itch extensively and be hard to control.

Pruritis (prue-rye-tis)

A skin condition that causes itching. The condition may influence a person to want to scratch the itch to relieve the concern, although doing so may put the body at an elevated risk of further harm.

Psoriasis (sore-eye-ah-sis)

A condition where skin cells build up in part of the body. The excess cells will produce scales and itchy patches on the skin. Dryness may also develop in the area. The condition may develop around many areas on the body, although this can be noticed particularly near the scalp. An infection may trigger psoriasis, although cold conditions may also be a factor. Topical treatments designed to clear the skin and to prevent skin cells from growing quickly may be applied to the impacted area.

Purpura (pur-pur-ah)

A series of red or purple spots that develop on the skin. These spots will not blanch or become white when you apply pressure. The spots are triggered by bleeding conditions under the skin and may be due to vascular or coagulation issues.

Purulent (pur-ue-lint)

Relating to pus.

PUVA

Psoralen ultraviolet A. This is a light therapy material. The drug will become active after it is exposed to the UVA light. This may help treat psoriasis, although other skin-related conditions may be treated by the light.

Pyoderma (pie-oh-dur-mah)

A skin disease that has pus. The condition may involve an ulcer or other conditions where the skin develops pus.

Rash

A series of spots that develop on the skin. The rash may have a bright red texture and may include several areas around the skin. The eruption is usually temporary, although it may reappear at times depending on the patient's skin quality.

Rhytidectomy (rie-tid-eck-toe-mee)

A face-lift procedure. The plastic surgery treatment involves the skin being lifted upward and old tissue near the scalp being removed. The process is to reduce the intensity of wrinkles on the face.

Rosacea (rose-a-sha)

A form of acne that develops in adults. The facial skin becoming red and may include a blushing or flushing appearance. Some pimples may form or swollen red bumps may be paired with some slightly visible blood vessels. The condition may become worse if not treated. Antibiotics are required to control the effects. Women are at an elevated risk of developing the issue.

Scabies (scay-bees)

Itching on the skin. This is caused by a mite that burrows into the skin and causes irritation in the tissue. The concern may become worse at night.

Scar

A permanent mark that appears after a wound heals. The scar is formed due to dead skin cells building up in the area of the wound. This could also be due to the blood flow to that part of the body not being healthy. Some scars may be reduced in intensity, although this would require extra topical treatments or laser solutions that target the deepest layers of skin.

Scleroderma (sk-lair-oh-dur-ma)

Crest syndrome. The skin because tight due to swelling. This may be noticed in the joint tissues. Joint pains can develop as an elevated response to cold conditions. Medications may be required to prevent the condition from developing and spreading to other parts of the body, especially to organs where the condition may become life-threatening.

Sebaceous Glands (see-bay-shus)

A series of small organs that are found in the dermis. The glands include ducts that open in a hair follicle and may go on the surface of the skin. A gland will produce sebum, an oily compound that lubricates the body. The gland may become clogged if not treated properly, thus resulting in acne.

Seborrhea (seb-or-ee-ah)

Also known as dandruff when this occurs on the scalp. Seborrhea causes a red rash with white scales developing in the impacted area. The rash produces scaly patches and will trigger white bits of skin coming off of the area. Medicated creams or shampoos may be required to treat the condition. Dandruff produced may be difficult to cover in some cases.

Sebum (see-bum)

The oily compound produced by the sebaceous glands. Sebum includes fat, keratin, and various compounds that are produced by cells and left behind after they evolve.

SLE

System lupus erythematosus. This is another term for lupus.

SPF

Skin protection factor. This is a measure of how well a sunscreen can protect the skin from UVB rays. The protection is required to prevent the development of sunburn, skin cancer, and other types of damage that may impact the skin. A higher SPF number will block a greater number of UVB rays. SPF 30 will block about 97% of UVB rays, and SPF 15 will block around 93% of those rays.

Squamous (skwa-mis)

Featuring scales.

Squamous Cell Carcinoma

Skin cancer. Unusual squamous cells will grow on the body. Areas that have been directly impacted by ultraviolet or UV rays will be more likely to experience SCC. The condition is more likely to develop in those who regularly use tanning beds. SCC may also impact the lungs as a form of lung cancer, although this is not as common as the skin-based condition.

Steatoma (stee-ah-toe-ma)

A cyst or tumor found in the sebaceous gland.

Subcutaneous (sub-cue-tain-ee-us)

Under the skin. This term refers mainly to the process of applying medication. The application works between the dermis and epidermis.

Sunburn

An injury on the skin due to excess exposure to sunlight or sunlamps. The burn develops due to the body taking in more ultraviolet light than what it can handle. The condition produces a red and painful surface on the skin. Blistering may develop in some cases. The pains involved become worse when a person touches the area. The condition may relieve on its own in a few days, although some pain relievers and topical agents may be applied to control the symptoms. A person who repeatedly gets sunburns may be at an elevated risk of developing skin cancer.

Sycosis (sigh-coe-sis)

Inflammation in the hair follicles around the face. The inflammation develops in hair that produces a beard. A bacterial infection will trigger the condition. This may also occur in other hair follicles, although this is more likely to develop in the facial area.

TEN

Topic epidermal necrolysis. A condition that involves the skin experiencing a severe reaction to certain treatments or compounds. This may trigger flu-like symptoms.

Tinea (tin-ee-ah)

A skin infection. This is a fungal condition that can be jock itch or athlete's foot. Excess moisture in the tissues may develop. People who are physically active and do not allow their bodies to air out or be washed off properly may be at a higher risk of developing tinea-related issues.

Ultraviolet

UV light. This is a form of light that has a wavelength of 10 to 400 nanometers. This is not visible light, but it appears mainly in the light produced by the sun. Excess exposure to UV light can cause sunburn and other skin issues. The UV light may also be linked to the development of many skin cancers and other conditions.

Ungual (un-gool)

Relating to the nails.

Unguis (un-gwee-ss)

A nail.

Urticaria (ur-ti-care-ee-ah)

Hives. A series of bumps or plaques called wheals may develop on the skin. Swelling occurs with skin welts developing in many patterns. This may be triggered by exposure to allergens or some medicines. Hives may produce itching and irritation. Antihistamines may be administered to reduce the intensity of the condition, although the condition may disappear on its own after a few days or weeks. Urticaria is chronic if the welts appear for at least six weeks at a time and consistently over a few months or years.

Verrucae (vair-ue-cay)

A plantar wart that develops on the soles of the feet or near the toe.

Vitiligo (vit-il-i-goe)

A chronic condition that causes white patches to develop around the skin. The patches may develop in various parts around the skin and can eventually cause the person's skin to be completely white. The vitiligo may be caused by genetics, although the death of melanocytes that produce the skin's pigment may also be a factor. The areas where vitiligo will develop around the body will be random and may cause significant or noticeable white spots to develop.

Wart

A benign growth. Also called verruca Vulgaris. The virus can impact the dermis and cause the development of a wart. The human papillomavirus or HPV may be a factor. Warts are likely to grow on the hands and feet, although they may develop on the genitals. The tissues produced will be thick and hard and may produce feelings of soreness. Warts can be contagious. Topical medications are recommended, although some procedures may also be conducted in a clinic to help remove warts if they are too prominent.

Weal (wheel)

A bump produced on the skin due to a blow. The area is red and can itch. The bump will disappear after a few hours, although the timeframe varies based on the intensity of the injury.

Wheal (wheel)

Swelling on the skin that develops due to an insect bite. This is similar to a weal.

Xeroderma (zer-oh-dur-mah)

A disease triggered by the skin being too dry. The condition develops mainly due to exposure to UV rays.

Prefixes

cutane/o   skin

derm/o   skin

derma	skin
dermat/o	skin
epitheli/o	epithelium
eschar/o	scab
follicul/o	follicle or cavity
hidr/o	sweat
lip/o	fat or lipid
melan/o	black or dark in tone
myc/o	fungus
onych/o	nail; this may be for either the finger or toe
pachy	thick
papul/o	papule or pimple
pil/o	hair
psor/o	itching
py/o	pus
rhytid/o	wrinkle
seb/o	sebum or oil; this may also be fatty deposits in the skin
squam/o	scaly
trich/o	hair
ungu/o	nail
xer/o	dry

Chapter 6 – Lymphatic System

The lymphatic system is a vital part of the immune system. The lymphatic system involves a series of vessels that will handle lymph functions. The lymph fluids in the body will drain from the body's tissues and into the blood. The fluids move towards the heart. The system controls difficult conditions and other problems that might affect the body.

This chapter includes details on how different conditions may be controlled by the lymphatic system. The chapter also includes information on various conditions relating to blood and how the body may be at risk of harm including conditions that may cause impairments to the immune system. The conditions are referred to by their abbreviations when applicable, as these are the terms that the conditions are often referenced by in most studies.

AIDS

Acquired immunodeficiency syndrome. The condition develops due to an infection of HIV or the human immunodeficiency virus. The T-cells in the body are not produced normally and prevent the immune system from functioning properly. The condition can cause muscle wasting and fatigue and eventually lead to death. The condition may be transmitted between people through sex or through sharing certain drugs or needles.

Adenitis (ad-in-eye-tis)

Inflammation in a lymph node that produces swelling.

Adenoid (ad-en-oid)

A series of lymph nodes on the posterior wall.

Adenoma (ad-en-oh-ma)

A benign tumor. The tumor is formed from glandular structures found in the epithelial tissue.

Adenovirus (ad-en-oh-vie-rus)

A virus that causes conjunctivitis, upper respiratory tract infections, and cystitis among other infections.

ALL

Acute lymphocytic leukemia. A blood cancer that develops in the bone marrow and influences white blood cells. A bone marrow cell will develop DNA errors and eventually divide causing the lymph nodes to become larger. The condition is common among children who experience cancers.

Allergen

A substance that causes a person to become overly sensitive to certain things.

AML

Acute myelogenous leukemia. The blood develops excess myeloid cells. The white blood cells are not appropriately mature. The condition can cause easy bruising and will eventually inhibit the development of new blood cells.

Antinuclear Antibody

Also called an ANA. A test that helps identify any possible autoimmune disorders. The test identifies if there are autoantibodies in the blood. A positive test may suggest that there are antibodies, but this may also indicate that a person has a disease. A full analysis of the patient's blood will have to be examined to identify if there is a concern with the immune system.

Anaphylaxis (an-ah-fil-ax-is)

An immune system reaction that develops when a person encounters an antigen. This often relates to when a person is in contact with a food-related allergen. The condition could be fatal depending on its intensity.

Antibiotic (an-tee-by-ot-ick)

A protein that is provided in a drug form. The protein is produced by blood plasma cells and will respond to antigens and other infections. The compound destroys bacteria, viruses, and toxins.

Antibody (an-tee-bo-dee)

A molecule form in immunoglobulin. The compound is produced in lymphoid tissue and will attack an antigen.

Antifungal (an-tee-fun-gull)

A drug that destroys fungi.

Antigen (an-te-gin)

A compound that is identified by the immune system and will lead to an immune reaction. The antigen may be a type of food or other natural material.

Antiviral (an-tee-vie-rul)

A compound that destroys a virus. The drug may also prevent the virus from replicating.

ARC

AIDS-related complex. This refers to the symptoms of a person who has been infected with HIV but has not developed the AIDS virus. The condition may involve swollen lymph glands among other concerns, although those risks might become more significant depending on the condition and how it develops.

ATL

Adult T-cell leukemia. May also be written as ATLL. Cancer that impacts the T-cells within the immune system.

Autoantibody (aw-toe-an-tee-bod-ee)

An antibody that responds to self-antigens in an organism that produced these compounds.

Autoantigens (aw-toe-an-te-gins)

Tissues that can interact with autoantibodies to produce immune responses.

Autoimmune (aw-toe-im-une)

A condition where the immune system triggers a response against tissues within the body, including healthy tissues.

Autoimmune Disorder

A name for a condition where a person's immune system attacks healthy cells.

Autoimmunity

A process where the immune system responds to its own tissue. The process triggers an autoimmune disorder.

Bacilli (bah-sil-ee)

A bacterium with a rod shape. The bacterium will trigger disease if enough of this compound is found.

Bacteria

A single cell compound.

CA

A possible abbreviation that may be used to describe cancer. The type of cancer should be identified and written before the CA.

Candidiasis (can-did-ee-ah-sis)

An infection that develops in wet skin areas. This is a yeast infection. The condition may develop due to the immune system being too weak or as a result of a person using antibiotics longer than necessary or at the wrong times.

Carcinogen (car-sin-oh-gin)

A compound that may trigger the development of some cancers.

Carcinoma (car-sin-oh-ma)

A cancerous disease where skin cells mutate.

Cervical Cancer

A condition where cancerous cells develop in the cervix. The condition mostly develops in older women. A Pap test is required to identify the development of cervical cancer in the female body. The condition may not have any symptoms.

Chemotherapy

A process where chemical compounds are used in the treatment of cancer and other conditions. The medications may be administered orally or intravenously. The chemotherapy agents will vary.

CLL

Chronic lymphocytic leukemia. Cancer involves B cells, which are white blood cells, mutating and eventually spreading to many parts of the body. The condition develops in older persons and can include fatigue and bruising and swelling in the lymph nodes.

CML

Chronic myeloid leukemia. The blood cancer that develops in the bone marrow due to a random chromosome mutation. The condition occurs mainly in older adults and can cause easy bleeding, fatigue, and unplanned or excessive weight loss.

CSD

Cat scratch disease or fever. The condition may develop due to a scratch or bite from a cat. The lymph nodes will become infected. The condition may produce red bumps around the skin and swelling in the lymph nodes near the injury. Although the condition may go away on its own, antibiotics may help reduce the effects.

Cytokines (sigh-toe-kins)

Compounds that are produced by immune system cells to convey information between one another.

Cytomegalovirus (sigh-toe-may-gah-loe-v-eye-rus)

Also known as CMV. The virus is related to the herpes virus. The condition will trigger cold sores in those who are infected. The issue may be identified by a blood test to review the IgG and IgM antibodies to identify the concern. Pneumonia will develop in those who have weakened immune systems.

Dengue (den-gee)

A disease that is transmitted by a bite from the infected Aedes mosquito. The condition may cause a fever and intense pain.

DPT

Diphtheria, pertussis, and tetanus vaccine.

EBV

Epstein-Barr virus. A condition that causes infectious mononucleosis.

ELISA

Enzyme-linked immunosorbent assay. A test that uses an enzyme in the body to identify the antibodies that may be present in the body. This may identify possible immune system and lymphatic issues in the body.

Epitope (ep-ee-taupe)

A spot on an antigen that will interact with antibodies.

GVHD

Graft-versus-host disease. Also known as runt disease. The condition involves bone marrow or stem cells that are transmitted to a patient through a donor. The cells will attack a person's immune system. The condition may develop when a person has gone through a transfusion or transplant and the new compound in one's body is not working properly.

Herpes

An infection that develops due to the herpes simplex virus. Type I may impact the mouth and produce cold sores around the region. Type II will influence the genital region and generate the same types of sores.

HIV

Human immunodeficiency virus. A condition that may be transferred through sexual intercourse or the sharing of medications or needles. The illness will influence the body's ability to control infections. The issue weakens the immune system and may lead to AIDS if the concern is not treated. Anti-retroviral therapy or ART will help slow the development of HIV and will also prevent the development of secondary infections in the body.

Hodgkin's Lymphoma

A lymphoma that develops in the lymph nodes. The condition may occur due to a lymph node becoming enlarged.

Hypersensitivity

When a person's immune system conducts an improper or excessive response to an antigen.

Immunity

The body's natural protection from diseases, particularly infectious ones.

Immunization

A process that gives the body the ability to resist diseases.

Immunoglobulin (im-you-noe-glob-you-lin)

A protein found in the serum and cells in the body's immune system. The proteins operate as antibodies.

Immunosuppressant

A drug that prevents the immune system from responding. The drug may work when attempting to clear an infection, although the drug may be too dangerous if used for too long or at the wrong time.

Immunotherapy

A process where the immune system is adjusted to treat a disease.

Interferon (in-tur-fear-on)

A small protein that is produced by T cells, fibroblasts, and other cells. The protein is produced as a response to a viral infection or another outside threat to the body.

Kaposi Sarcoma (kap-oe-see)

Cancer that produces lesions on the body including lesions around the lymph nodes and other organs. Cancer may include improperly formed blood cells and vessels.

Lymph (lim-f)

The fluid produced in the lymphatic system. The fluid includes white blood cells and will drain the lymphatic system into the bloodstream.

Lymph Node

A part of the body that will filter substances that move through the lymphatic fluid. The nodes may include the white blood cells needed to control the development of the nodes.

Lymphadenitis (lim-pha-den-eye-tis)

Inflammation in the lymph node.

Lymphadenopathy (lim-pha-den-aw-pa-thee)

Inflammation in the lymph node that results in the tissue becoming enlarged.

Lymphangiectasis (lim-fan-ject-a-sis)

When the lymph nodes become enlarged.

Lymphangioma (lim-fan-ge-oh-ma)

A change in the lymphatic system. This includes a congenital impact that keeps the system from operating properly.

Lymphangiosarcoma (lim-fan-ge-oh-sar-koe-mah)

A malignant tumor that develops from the endothelial cells in the lymph nodes.

Lymphedema (lim-feh-dee-mah)

Edema caused by the lymph nodes not working properly. The areas may be obstructed and unable to drain properly. The condition may develop in the arms after some surgical treatments.

Lymphocele (lim-foe-cell)

A cystic mass that includes lymph tissue.

Lymphocytosis (lim-foe-sigh-toe-sis)

An increase in the number of lymphocytes in the blood.

Lymphoma (lim-foe-mah)

A rise in the number of lymphocytes found in the blood.

Lymphoma (lim-foe-mah)

A condition where lymphocytes are impacted and become cancerous. The condition will cause the lymph nodes to work improperly. The issue may cause enlarged lymph nodes and unplanned weight loss as well as fatigue.

Lymphopenia (lim-foe-pen-ee-ah)

A decline in the number of lymphocytes in the blood.

Macrophage (mack-roe-phayge)

A white blood cell in the immune system. The cell will remove unwanted cells including any cells that might cause illnesses. Any debris left over by the cell will also be eliminated by the macrophage.

Malaria (mal-air-e-ah)

An illness caused by an infected mosquito bite. The issue can cause chills, flu-like symptoms, and diarrhea. The condition is more common in underdeveloped parts of the world.

Mammography (mam-og-ra-phee)

An examination of the breast tissue through low-energy x-rays. The test identifies cases of breast cancer and may detect the condition before it becomes more difficult to treat.

Metastasis (met-ah-stay-sis)

When cancer spreads to another part of the body. This includes a section of the body that had not dealt with cancer in the past.

Myosarcoma (my-oh-sar-koe-ma)

A malignant tumor in the muscle. The tissue may cause a muscle to weaken and to develop a persistent cramping sensation.

Osteosarcoma (os-te-oh-sar-koe-ma)

A form of cancer that creates immature bone structures. The issue may be found at the ends of long bones and especially will form in the knee area. The condition develops mainly in younger persons. The issue can cause intense pain and swelling in the impacted area and may also cause problems where the body might weaken.

Parasite (pear-a-sight)

An organism that will travel to another organism. A parasite may transfer an illness or other condition to a person who is infected. The parasite may enter through the blood or skin.

Preleukemia

A condition where the blood or bone marrow appears to be developing the early stages of leukemia. The condition has not become prominent, nor it is causing the symptoms of leukemia immediately. Proper treatment is required to ensure the concern is treated so the risk of leukemia is minimal.

Rabies (ray-bees)

A viral infection transmitted through the saliva of an infected animal. The animal bite may trigger a fever, muscle spasms, paralysis, and possibly death. The condition may develop throughout the world, although it is most prominent in Australia, China, India, and much of Africa. Animals that may have rabies include raccoons, bats, foxes, and some cats and dogs that are not appropriately vaccinated against the condition.

Rickettsia (rick-it-see-ah)

Bacteria surrounded by a layer of protein. The bacteria may be transmitted to humans through various insects, particularly spiders or scorpions. People who are infected develop conditions such as typhus, Lyme disease, or Rocky Mountain spotted fever.

Rubella (rue-bel-ah)

Also known as German measles. A viral disease that enters the respiratory tract and will spread to the lymphatic system. A rash will develop throughout the body. The lymph nodes in the neck will also become enlarged. The condition mostly impacts children and young adults. The condition may cause deafness.

Sarcoidosis (sar-koid-oh-sis)

Inflammation that develops through the lymphatic system. The inflammation develops in the lymph glands and lungs, although it may also spread to other tissues in the body.

Granulomas that include enlarged cells can develop. The inflammation may last for a few weeks and can go away on its own, but other situations may last for years and could produce organ failure unless the condition is treated soon.

Sarcoma (sar-koe-mah)

Cancer in the connective tissues. This is a soft tissue condition that will impact fat, muscle, cartilage, and other soft tissues within the body. Cancer will develop in the bone structure and spread to the soft tissues. Some lumps may be found in parts of the body that have been impacted. The symptoms will vary based on where in the body the condition has developed.

Scrofula (skro-fue-lah)

Tuberculosis that impacts the lymph nodes, especially the nodes in the neck.

Spleen

An organ found near the stomach. The organ will filter blood in the immune system and will recycle old red blood cells. White blood cells and platelets may be stored in the tissue. A patient may live without a spleen, although that person may be at an elevated risk of developing infections due to the lack of the organ.

Splenectomy (splen-eck-toe-mee)

The removal of the spleen. The entire organ or a part of it is removed.

Splenitis (spleen-eye-tis)

Inflammation in the spleen.

Splenomegaly (splen-oh-may-gal-ee)

When the spleen becomes enlarged.

Staphylococci (staff-ill-oh-cock-eye)

Also known as staph. The bacteria have a spherical appearance and will develop in a series of small clusters. The bacteria will prevent various infections, although the bacteria itself may become infected if not treated properly.

TAT

Tetanus antitoxin. The compound is administered when a person experiences a penetrating wound that could become contaminated with soil. The antitoxin helps to treat immediate risks, although the patient should seek further attention to prevent the issue from becoming worse.

Tetanus (tet-nus)

Also known as lockjaw. The condition is caused by the body contracting Clostridium bacteria through a deep cut. This includes a cut that may happen by stepping on a nail. The bacterial infection can cause muscle spasms including intense pains in the neck and jaw areas and could be deadly if left untreated.

Thymectomy (thy-meck-toe-mee)

The removal of the thymus gland.

Thymocytes (thy-moe-cites)

Lymphocytes that develop in the thymus.

Thymoma (thy-moe-mah)

A tumor that develops in the epithelial cells in the thymus. The condition may cause difficulties in swallowing and pains in the chest.

Thymus (thy-mus)

An organ that produces T lymphocytes. The organ will help to get the cells to work in the immune system. The organ is found in the chest area.

TNF

Tumor necrosis factor. The TNF is a cell-signaling protein that triggers systemic inflammation and may lead to the general acute reaction to certain conditions.

Tonsillectomy (ton-sil-eck-toe-mee)

The surgical removal of a tonsil. Both tonsils may be removed in the process.

Tonsils (ton-sills)

A pair of tissues near the back part of the throat. These are lymphatic tissues that will filter out various compounds in the body.

Toxoplasmosis (tocks-oh-plas-moe-sis)

A parasitic disease caused by the Toxoplasma gondii parasite. The condition may not cause any symptoms at the beginning, but this may lead to some flu-like symptoms after a while. The condition is dangerous and potentially fatal to pregnant women and those with weakened immune systems. The condition may be spread mainly in those who are in contact with cat fecal matter or contaminated food.

Vaccination

A process where a vaccine is administered to the patient's body.

Vaccine

A material that includes microorganisms that have been engineered to prevent an infection. Vaccines are produced to control the body's lymphatic system to respond to any possible materials that could possibly cause such infections.

Varicella (vair-e-cel-ah)

Also known as chickenpox. The condition is triggered by the varicella-zoster virus. The issue will cause an itchy rash to develop and can produce blisters on the skin. The condition may be contagious to anyone who has never had the disease or has not been vaccinated to prevent the issue. The virus may also be reactivated later in life, thus producing the herpes zoster rash.

WBC

White blood count. This is a measure of the number of white blood cells in the blood. A minimal number suggests that a person has an immune disorder. An excess number may indicate that a person has a condition relating to the production of bone marrow.

Prefixes

anti	against or working opposite of
carcin/o	cancerous
immune/o	immune or relating to the immune system
leukocyt/o	white blood cell
lien/o	spleen
lymph/o	lymph
lymphaden/o	lymph node
lymphangia/o	lymph vessel
onc/o	soft tumor

phag/o	eating or swallowing
sarc/o	connective tissue
scirrh/o	hard tumor
tonsill/o	tonsil

Chapter 7 – Muscular System

The muscular system refers to the muscles in the human body. Many of the terms involved with the muscular system focus on how the system may be negatively influenced based on how well different functions in the muscles may operate and how they are controlled properly.

Many conditions listed are either voluntary or involuntary motions. Voluntary motions refer to ones that a person is capable of doing without help. Involuntary motions are ones that a person is unable to control.

Some of the terms involved focus on the axis of the body. The axis is a reference to the line on which the body rotates. The movements in the body take place in a plane along an axis. This includes an axis that is horizontal, vertical, or diagonal.

Abduction

A process when a limb is moved from the midline or axis of the body.

Achilles Tendon

The area near the back heel. The tendon connects the muscles in the back part of the calf to the calcaneus or heel bone.

Actomyosin (ack-toe-my-oh-sin)

A complex of actin and myosin that develops in the human muscle tissue. This is a contractile material that will support the functionality of the muscle and its ability to be active.

Adduction

When a limb moves towards the midline or axis of the body.

Adductor (ad-uck-tor)

A muscle that allows a body part to move towards the axis of the body.

Adhesion

Scar tissues that develop in the body following a surgery.

ADL

Activities of daily living. A doctor's report may include an analysis of the ADL to identify how active a person is to identify if there are certain physical conditions that might be impacting what they can do.

Aerobics (air-oh-bix)

Strenuous exercise activities. The exercise helps improves upon the cardiovascular and respiratory systems.

Anconeus (an-con-ee-us)

A triangular muscle that develops under the elbow. The muscle helps support the forearm tissue.

Antispasmodic (an-tee-spas-mod-ik)

A drug that will treat smooth muscle spasms in the digestive system or urinary tract. The drug focuses on involuntary movements.

Astasia (as-tay-sha)

When a person is unable to stand or sit without assistance. The problem may develop in the muscles, although this could be for reasons beyond physical causes.

Ataxia (at-ax-e-ah)

An inability to coordinate one's voluntary muscle movements. Ataxia does not develop due to muscle weakness.

Atonic (a-ton-ik)

When a muscle does not attain its regular tone or strength level.

Atrophy (at-roe-fee)

When the muscle wastes. The muscle tissue will be smaller in size, usually due to poor nutrition, a lack of physical activity, or an autoimmune disorder.

Baclofen (back-loe-fin)

A drug that relaxes the muscle and decreases muscle spasms. This may be offered under brand names like Gablofen and Lioresal.

Ballism (ball-izm)

Unusual movements of the limbs.

Biceps (bi-seps)

A muscle that extends from the shoulder joint to the elbow. The word 'biceps' may also refer to any muscle that has two head surfaces.

Bradykinesia (bray-de-kin-ee-sha)

Slow body movement. This is when a person experiences weakness and tremors in the body and some rigidity in movement. The condition may be a sign of Parkinson's disease.

Buttocks

One of the two fleshy areas around the lower posterior part of the trunk or hip. The buttocks consist of fats and gluteal muscles.

Carpal Tunnel Syndrome

A condition when a person experiences numbness and pain in the hand. This may be intense tensions that are not easily relieved by some medications. The condition is associated with many repetitive tasks in the workplace, particularly working on a keyboard. Wrist injuries and rheumatoid arthritis can aggravate CTS. Pregnancy may also trigger CTS.

Chronic Fatigue Syndrome

Also known as CFS. A condition when a person experiences fatigue that cannot be relieved with rest. The issue may be a hormonal concern or could be a sign of problems with the body's muscles.

Circumduction (sir-cum-duc-shun)

A movement of a limb that extends from one joint to the next.

Contracture (con-trak-sure)

A condition where elastic tissues are replaced by inelastic tissues. This is a shortening of a muscle or joint. The condition develops due to hypertonic spasticity in a certain muscle area and may be noticed in conditions like cerebral palsy.

Cool Down

The process by which the body's heart rate, blood pressure, and body temperature drop after an exercise. The effort is progressive, although it can take a few hours for the body to fully return to its resting rate.

Dantrolene (dan-troe-lean)

A muscle relaxant often offered as Dantrium or Ryanodex. The condition treats stiffness and spasms including conditions that are produced by cerebral palsy, multiple sclerosis, or other conditions that negatively impact the muscles.

Deltoid (del-toid)

A triangular muscle in the shoulder. The tissue's function is to flex and extend the arm's position.

Dorsiflexion (dor-sif-lex-shun)

The movement of the ankle joint. The movement brings the dorsal or top part of the foot towards the shin.

DTR

Deep tendon reflex. The movement helps stretch the muscles and is used to test how well the spinal cord works. The reflex is examined to identify the possibility of a neuromuscular condition developing in the body.

Dyskinesia (dis-ken-ee-sha)

Involuntary movements in the facial, trunk, and neck muscles among others. This may be problems trying to move the muscles. The concern is frequently associated with medication use.

Dystonia (dis-ton-ee-ah)

A disorder that involves involuntary muscle contractions. Muscle movements will cause slow movements or unusual body positions. The condition is repetitive in nature.

Dystrophy (dis-troe-fee)

A condition that results due to a part of the body not getting the necessary nutrition. The issue may impact the muscles.

Electromyography (e-lek-troe-my-oh-gra-fee)

A test to measure the electrical activities of the muscles. The activities are analyzed through a visual display. Electrodes are applied along the skin, although some may be added into the muscles. The electrical signals are analyzed based on muscle movements and how great response is produced. The EMG may assist in determining if certain movements are voluntary.

Extraocular Muscles (ex-tra-oc-u-lur)

The six muscles that control the eye movement and the levator palpebrae, the muscle that controls how eyelids move up and down. The muscles are analyzed to determine how well the muscles contract based on where the eye is positioned when a treatment is given.

Epicondylitis (ep-ik-on-dyl-eye-tis)

Tennis elbow. The condition occurs when the forearm is injured due to excessive use or a strain. The tendons in the forearm area can develop tears.

Epimysium (ep-ee-my-see-um)

The fibrous connective tissue that covers a skeletal muscle.

Ergonomics

Designs that help reduce the stress or injuries in the body. The ergonomics help keep injuries from developing as a result of muscles being overused. Bad posture problems may also be prevented, particularly ones relating to what happens when the body is made to repeatedly complete various tasks.

Extensor (ex-ten-sore)

A muscle that extends to another body part.

Fascia (fas-shah)

A layer of fibrous tissue. This is the connective tissue that surrounds muscles, nerves, and blood vessels.

Fasciitis (fash-eye-tis)

Inflammation of the fascia.

Fibromyalgia (fie-bro-my-al-jah)

Also known as fibrositis. The disorder produces musculoskeletal pain around the entire body. The condition occurs as fatigue and develops into a pain in the tissues. The brain may recognize pain signals stronger than what would be considered normal. The condition may be treated through medications or with efforts to reduce stress in the body in general.

Flexor

A muscle that allows a limb to bend

Ganglion Cyst (gang-le-on)

Also called a bible cyst. A swelling will develop on the covering of a tendon. The cyst has an appearance like a sac of liquid. The cyst includes a jellylike and sticky material that may feel firm or soft. The joints or tendons on the wrists and hands are where the condition is more likely to develop. The condition is benign and may go away on its own over a few weeks, although the condition can be removed or drained through a needle if necessary.

Heel Spur

A small bony outgrowth that appears on the lower end of the heel bone. This is a calcium deposit that builds up on the underside of the heel bone. The growth may go away on its own, although some therapy may be required. Surgery is not required for treating a heel spur in most cases.

Hemiparesis (hem-e-par-e-sis)

Paralysis or weakness on one side of the body. The condition may be triggered by a stroke or tumor, or physical trauma. The condition may be temporary.

Hemiplegia (hem-e-plee-gee-ah)

Paralysis on one side of the body.

Hernia (hur-nee-ah)

The protrusion of tissue or another structure that may go through a bone. This includes a tissue or organ that moves out from its normal position.

Hyperkinesia (high-per-kin-ee-sha)

Sudden involuntary movements in the body. These can develop at random throughout the body.

Hyperkinesis (high-pur-kin-ee-sis)

When muscles in the body move too often.

Hypnic Jerk (hip-nick)

A myoclonic twitch that develops when a person is asleep.

Hypotonia (high-poe-tone-ee-ah)

Floppy baby syndrome. The condition occurs when muscle tone is low. The muscle will not produce much tension to stretch, thus causing the muscle to become weak. The hypotonia condition may be noticed in children, hence the floppy baby syndrome name. This may also develop in older persons.

Impingement Syndrome

Swimmer's shoulder. A tendon frequently rubs along a shoulder blade. The condition causes fatigue in the body. Inflammation can occur as well as an elevated risk of injury to the area.

Intermittent Claudication

Muscle pains produced because there is not enough blood flowing in the body. The condition appears during exercise.

Intramuscular

When something takes place inside a muscle or when a drug is administered into the muscle tissue.

Intrinsic Muscle

A muscle where the origin and insertion occur in the same part or organ.

Isotonic Contraction

A muscle contraction that develops with a minimal change in the contraction force. This may also involve a shortening of the distance between the origin and insertion points. The maximal force of contraction will exceed the load on the muscle. This may be a concentric condition where the muscle shortens or an eccentric condition where the muscle lengthens.

Masseter Muscle

A thick muscle in the cheek that will close the jaw.

Muscular Dystrophy

Also called MD. An inherited disease that will cause muscle weakness and loss. There are more than 30 such inherited diseases that may be interpreted as MD. The specific disease contracted will vary based on the time in one's life when MD develops or the muscles that the condition will influence. The genetic condition will produce the loss of muscle mass and can cause the body to weaken over time. The most significant conditions may result in difficulty in breathing and swallowing.

Myalgia (my-al-jah)

Muscle pain. The pain may develop because of many issues including when a muscle or a series of muscles are stretched too far. The condition may disappear on its own with rest, although myalgia may be chronic in some cases. People who experience viral infections are more likely to regularly contract myalgia.

Myasthenia Gravis (my-as-thee-neea gra-viss)

An autoimmune disease triggered by the skeletal muscles becoming weak. The condition may be noticed by some muscles that are impacted drooping and being hard to control. A patient may develop double vision and troubles with swallowing. This includes difficulties with walking properly or normally.

Myocele (my-oh-cell)

A muscle substance that protrudes through a hole in a sheath.

Myoclonus (my-oh-clon-us)

The sudden movement of a muscle. A patient may develop a twitching sensation. Sudden contractions make up positive episodes of myoclonus. Brief contraction lapses are negative episodes.

Myofascial Release (my-oh-fa-shul)

A process that restores motions in tissues that are feeling pain. The process involves relaxing the muscles and using planned stretching. Myofascial release will relax muscles and improve upon how blood flows in the body. This may also enhance the lymphatic circulation in some areas.

Myogenic (my-oh-gen-ick)

A condition that develops in the muscles.

Myolysis (my-ole-eye-sis)

When muscle tissues break down.

Myoma (my-oh-ma)

Also known as fibroids. Myomas are benign tumors that consist mainly of muscle tissues. The myoma is unlike to develop in the cervix, although it may occur more likely in the uterus. Fibroids will trigger low back pain and may cause a woman's menstrual cycle to last longer than normal.

Myoparesis (my-oh-par-e-sis)

Weakness or paralysis in the muscle. This may also refer to a suture of muscle tissue.

Myositis (my-ohs-eye-tis)

Inflammation in a muscle or the tissue involved.

Myotonia (my-oh-tone-ee-ah)

A sudden muscle spasm that develops or muscular rigidity.

Myotonic (my-oh-ton-ick)

Relating to muscle tone.

Neuromuscular

A type of muscular disorder. The nerves that control voluntary muscles are affected.

NMJ

Neuromuscular junction. A synapse that develops between a motor neuron and a muscle fiber. Acetylcholine is released into the synapse when an action occurs. The event will trigger an appropriate result based on the sensations felt.

Nocturnal Myoclonus

Also known as periodic limb movement disorder. The patient experiences regular limb movements while asleep. The condition is not related to restless leg syndrome or RLS. The muscle movements that occur during sleep are involuntary and impact small muscles. The arms and legs may be influenced in some cases.

Oblique (ob-leek)

An outside muscle that supports the abdomen.

Obturator Muscle

The muscle that appears on the ischium and rim of the pubic. The muscle goes through the pelvic cavity. The tissue is needed to allow the thighs to rotate outward.

Paralysis (par-al-y-sis)

When the muscles are unable to function properly.

Paraplegia (pear-a-plea-gee-ah)

Paralysis that involves the legs. The condition may develop due to a spinal cord injury.

Pectoral (peck-taur-ul)

A muscle on the front part of the chest. The muscle surrounds the bones on the shoulder and upper arm areas. Pectoral is part of the human thorax.

Pectus Carinatum (peck-tus car-i-nay-tum)

A condition where the chest wall appears to thrust outward. The sternum cartilage may become excessive, thus causing the bulge. This may be called pigeon chest due to the bird-like appearance of the chest. This is a birth defect that may be treated by the use of a brace. A surgical procedure is necessary when the regular treatment process fails to correct the condition.

Pelvic Floor

Muscles along the bottom of the pelvic area. These include tissues under the perineum and pelvis. The muscles support the tissues and go from the pubic bone to the coccyx. The pelvic floor is important for women as it is the region of the body that is mainly involved in the child birthing process.

Plantar Fascitis (plan-tar fahs-eye-tis)

Also known as policeman's or postman's heel. Inflammation develops in the plantar fascia, a tissue that secures the hell bone to the toes. The inflammation results in intense pain in the heel area with the pain being worse in the morning. Physical therapy and steroid injections may help, although shoe inserts can also help. The irritation is more likely to develop among older persons.

Polymyositis (pol-e-my-oh-sigh-tis)

An inflammatory condition where the muscles and the blood vessels become inflamed due to cellular damage.

Pronation

Rotation of the foot while walking. Pronation is the foot rotating inward. The foot moves inward and does not stay straight when walking. This is the opposite of supination, where the foot moves outward. Appropriate footwear may be required to correct or reduce the intensity of the pronation or supination.

Pyomyositis (pie-oh-my-ohs-eye-tis)

A bacterial infection in the skeletal muscles. The condition may trigger pus-filled abscesses and is common in tropical areas, although it may also occur in other zones. The problem develops mainly in the larger skeletal muscle groups.

Quadriceps (quad-ri-seps)

A muscle in the thigh. The muscle is named for having a four-headed surface.

Quadriplegia (quad-ri-plea-jah)

Paralysis that is the loss of use of all the limbs and the torso. This may also involve the partial loss of the use of the tissues.

Rhabdomyoma (rab-doe-my-oh-ma)

A neoplasm that develops in striated muscle. The neoplasm is benign.

Rhabdomyosarcoma (rab-doe-my-oh-sar-coe-ma)

A malignant neoplasm that occurs in striated muscle.

RICE

A treatment process that may be used to relieve pains in the muscles. The process includes rest, ice to be applied on the surface, compression of the tissue, and elevation of the impacted area.

Rotator Cuff

A series of muscles and tendons that support the shoulder. The rotator cuff is used when moving the shoulder to keep the joint functional. The area may be torn or fatigued due to excess use.

RSI

Repetitive stress injury. The issue occurs due to the tissue being impacted.

Sarcocystosis (sar-coe-sis-toe-sis)

An infection in the striated muscle by a parasite. The condition may trigger vomiting, diarrhea, and muscle weakness. The most significant cases may result in paralysis.

Sarcopenia (sar-coe-pen-ee-ah)

A disease that develops as the body ages. The person may experience a loss in muscle mass and strength.

Sartorius (sar-taur-ee-us)

An anterior thigh muscle that is found from the pelvis to the calf.

Shin Splint

Small tears in the muscle and bone tissue in the body. The tears develop due to excess use in the shinbone area. The splint develops when muscles or tendons become overworked. This may develop among those who have been working harder to train their muscles and could be a concern to those who are trying to dramatically change their training routines.

Shivering

A shaking process. The body shivers when conditions are cold. The actions occur as a warm-blooded body aims to keep warm. As the body's temperature drops, the shivering reflex will be activated to keep the body comfortable, thus supporting homeostasis. The skeletal muscles may also shake in small movements, thus producing added warmth through the energy produced in the body.

Singultus (sin-gul-tus)

A condition known as hiccupping. The diaphragm experiences a spasm. This may be a response to foods consumed or from air moving through the area. The spasms may be temporary, although they can be chronic and may trigger some actions in brief periods depending on the intensity of the hiccups that occur.

Soleus (sol-ee-us)

A flat muscle in the calf.

Spasm

An involuntary muscular contraction. The muscle is unable to relax during a spasm. A mild twitch may develop in some cases, although some intense pains may occur depending on how sensitive the impacted area is. Spasms occur often in skeletal muscles and may be due to fatigue and dehydration or from lack of electrolytes in the body.

Striated Muscle (stree-ate-ed)

A skeletal muscle.

Spasmodic Torticollis (spas-moe-dik tor-ti-col-is)

A chronic condition where the neck will involuntarily turn left, right, up, or down. The condition may be called cervical dystonia. Multiple muscle tissues will move.

Sphincter (ss-fink-tur)

A small muscle at the end of the rectum and urinary tract. The muscle produces constrictions that allow wastes to pass through the body. The tissue will relax as necessary.

Sprain

An injury that develops when the fibers in a ligament are torn. The condition may heal on its own through rest and elevation, although the pains involved may be intense at times. The healing time will vary based on how intense the sprain is. The ankle, wrist, thumb, and knee are among the most common parts of the body that can develop sprains. A sprain may also be measured based on how intense it is. A grade one sprain will be slight stretching and can take up to two weeks to heal. A grade two sprain produces stiffness and irritation in the body and can take about four to six weeks to heal.

Tendinous (ten-din-is)

A condition that relates to tendons.

Tendon (ten-din)

A flexible tissue of fibrous collagen that connects a muscle to a bone.

Tensor (ten-sore)

A muscle that causes stretching or tension in a part of the body.

Tetany (tet-an-ee)

A condition where muscle spasms and cramps develop. Twitching may also occur. The issue develops because the body has a low blood calcium level or hypocalcemia. A blood test may be conducted to identify the calcium level and to determine if there is a problem.

Tibialis (tib-ee-al-is)

A muscle that appears around the upper part of the tibia. This is on the lateral or outside surface of the tibia. The muscle continues into the medial cuneiform and the first few metatarsal bones in the foot. The muscle helps adjust the foot's position with regards to the rest of the body.

Tonic

Referring to regular muscle tone.

Tremor

Shaking that occurs without warning.

Triceps (tri-seps)

A muscle with three heads. The triceps is a muscle on the back part of the upper arm that links to the forearm.

Prefixes

asthen	weakness
desm/o	ligament
ergo	energy
fasci/o	fascia
fibr/o	fiber
flex/o	flex
herni/o	hernia
kinesi/o	movement
lei/o	smooth
leiomy/o	smooth muscle
muscl/o	muscle
my/o	muscle
pyg/o	buttocks
rhabdomy/o	striated muscle
spasmo	spasm
sthen/o	strength
syndesm/o	ligament
tax/o	coordination
ten/o	tendon
tendin/o	tendon

ton/o   tension

Chapter 8 – Nervous System

The nervous system is a series of nerve cells and fibers that transmit nerve impulses between different parts of the body. The system ensures that many actions are supported by the body including sensory information that involves identifying what is happening within the body when attempting various physical activities.

The terms in this chapter focus on functions within the nervous system. This includes impairments and concerns that may develop due to improper activities within the nervous system. Many of these are concerns that may influence one's behavior or physical functionalities. In some cases, a person's intellectual development may be affected.

Accessory Nerve

A cranial nerve used for swallowing, speech, and various head and shoulder movements.

Acrophobia (ack-roe-foe-bee-a)

A fear of heights. The condition often triggers an elevated heart rate when a person notices something relating to being high up in the air.

Acupuncture (ack-ue-punk-ture)

An alternative form of medicine that focuses on relieving the nervous system. The treatment involves needles being applied around certain pathways on the nervous system. The effort helps allow energy to flow through the body's meridians, thus enhancing how the body can recover from various physical concerns.

Alzheimer's Disease (Alz-high-murz)

A condition where a person develops dementia to where one's behaviors become irrational or one's memory becomes impaired. This may result in some difficulties with thinking or performing routine actions.

ADD

Attention deficit disorder. This is a concern where a person becomes impulsive or hyperactive. This may cause a person to have a hard time paying attention to certain things or maintain focus.

ADHD

Attention deficit hyperactivity disorder. ADHD is the same thing as ADD.

Adjustment Disorder

When a person is unable to properly respond to a certain stressful occasion.

Adrenergic Fibers (ad-ren-ur-jic)

Nerve fibers that allow movements and sensations to travel through a synapse. These fibers respond to an impulse that the body may develop.

Adrenergic Neurons

Neurons that operate from the production of epinephrine.

Affect (a-fect)

The reaction that a person has to a thought or experience.

Agnosia (ag-no-see-a)

An inability to understand the importance of some kind of stimulation. This may include being unable to recognize the issue.

Akinetic Mutism (mu-tizm)

A concern where a person is silent and inactive while not engaging in any voluntary motor actions in spite of the person being alert of their surroundings.

Alexia (al-ecks-ee-a)

An inability to read something in spite of being able to write. The person is unable to recognize words and letters. This may be a sign of Alzheimer's or another degenerative condition.

Alprazolam (al-pra-zoe-lam)

A common medication used for the treatment of anxiety or panic issues. The condition is available commercially under the Xanax name.

Amnesia (am-knee-shah)

A condition where a person loses their memory due to an emotional event or from brain injury. The condition is not permanent.

Amphetamine (am-fet-a-meen)

A drug that stimulates the central nervous system. The drug enhances the person's alertness.

Amyotrophic Lateral Sclerosis (eh-me-oh-troe-phic lat-ur-ul sklur-oh-sis)

Also called ALS or may be referred to as Lou Gehrig's Disease. A condition where neurons deteriorate over time, eventually weakening the muscles and destroying the body's natural physical functions.

Analgesia (an-el-gess-ee-ah)

When a person does not feel pain or feels less pain than usual.

Analgesic (an-el-jeess-ik)

A drug that relieves pain.

Anesthesia (an-es-thee-see-ah)

When a person no longer feels anything. This includes not feeling pain. The process is induced before any surgical treatments are performed.

Anesthetic (an-es-thet-ik)

A medication that causes a person to lose sensation. The medication is used to treat pain and is especially needed prior to a surgical procedure. A general anesthetic may be given to treat any part of the body. A local anesthetic focuses on a very specific area on the body and numbs only that area.

Anhedonia (an-he-done-ee-ah)

An inability to feel pleasure. This is a concern found in some psychotic disorders.

Anomia (an-oh-mee-ah)

An inability to name things that one might normally be able to identify.

Anticonvulsant (an-tee-con-vul-sint)

A drug that prevents or reduces the intensity of seizures.

Antidepressant (an-tee-dee-press-int)

A drug that controls the signs of depression.

Antidromic (an-tee-droe-mick)

Nerve impulses that are transmitted in a different direction than usual.

Antipsychotic (an-tee-sigh-kot-ik)

A drug that treats significant mental conditions. The drug is a tranquilizer. Such drugs may be prescribed for the treatment of significant concerns relating to paranoia or hallucinations.

Antisocial (an-tee-soe-shul)

A personality trait where a person does not have any respect for individual rights or other rules. This may include a person who refuses to participate with others in various activities.

Anxiety

A general feeling of dread in spite of there being no stimuli supporting this feeling.

Apathy

When a person does not feel any emotion.

Aphasia (ah-fay-sha)

An inability to comprehend language or speech.

Apraxia (ap-racks-ee-ah)

A disorder where a person is unable to make proper decisions or movements. This may be caused by cerebral impairment.

Aptitude Test

A test that identifies a person's intellect or ability to learn.

Aquaphobia

A general fear of water. This may be noticed during an attempt to try to treat a person with water.

Arachnoid (ar-ack-noid)

A membrane that covers the brain and spinal cord.

Arachnoiditis (ar-ack-noid-eye-tis)

Inflammation in the arachnoid. This may cause intense pain and some neurological impairments.

Arousal

A condition where a person becomes alert or overly alert after being stimulated. Arousal often refers to sexual feelings.

Asperger's Syndrome (as-pur-gurz)

A developmental condition where a person lacks social interactivity. This includes cases where a person engages in the same patterns of behavior. A person may also be impaired in language or the ability to communicate with others. In some cases, the condition may include an unusual fixation on certain activities or interests.

Assertiveness

When a person is overly insistent in behaviors. This may be a sign of a person being overly protective of the self or fearful.

Astrocyte (as-trough-cite)

A star-shaped cell that is found in the central nervous system.

Astrocytoma (as-troe-sigh-toe-mah)

A tumor found in the brain that comes from astrocytes. The tumor will not spread outside of the brain, but it may impair how the brain functions.

Autism (aw-tizm)

A developmental condition where a person experiences substantial social and communicative disabilities. This includes an inability to communicate with others properly or an inability to have proper behaviors in most public situations.

Autonomic Nervous System

A segment of the nervous system that focuses on involuntary functions. This includes the enteric, parasympathetic, and sympathetic nervous systems. The name includes the word autonomic, which means able to function without an outside influence involved.

Autophagia (aw-toe-fay-gee-ah)

A condition where a person consistently bites their own flesh.

Aversion Therapy

A treatment where a person is kept from engaging in unwanted behaviors by being regularly exposed to unpleasant effects surrounding those behaviors. The concept is designed to encourage people to stop engaging in behaviors that might be harmful.

Avoidance

When a person emotionally tries to avoid an experience that they do not want to have.

Axon (ax-on)

A nerve fiber that produces impulses that leads away from the neuron cells.

BAC

Blood alcohol content. This is a measure of the concentration of alcohol in a person's body. A person with a BAC of at least 0.08% may be interpreted as being impaired and could be arrested for driving while intoxicated. An exceptionally high BAC may cause a person to be at risk of brain damage.

Barbiturate (bar-bich-ur-eight)

A sedative that weakens the central nervous system. The drug can also reduce the patient's blood pressure, respiratory rate, and temperature.

Basal Ganglia (bay-sul gang-lee-ah)

A small series of components in the brain. The components are connected to the brainstem, cerebral cortex, and thalamus. The tissues help control motor functions like eye movements. These parts may also influence emotional responses and general cognition.

Bell's Palsy

A condition that impacts the seventh cranial nerve. One side of the face becomes paralyzed. The condition is often temporary.

Benzocaine (ben-zoe-caine)

An anesthetic that is applied as topical pain relief. This is found under the Orajel name among other brand names, although a hospital may use a stronger concentration of the drug for more intense situations.

Bipolar Disorder

A condition where a person may develop extreme mood swings. These include manic and depressive episodes.

Brain

A segment in the central nervous system that controls functions relating to the body's production and support. The brain is situated within the cranium.

Carotid Ultrasonography

An ultrasound test that reviews the carotid arteries. The test investigates for blood clots and other issues that may directly influence the brain's natural functions.

Catatonia (cat-ah-tone-e-ah)

A condition where a person becomes mute and immobile due to the muscles in a part of the body becoming rigid and impossible to move.

Cauda Equina (cau-dah eq-wee-na)

The lower segment of the spinal cord where the lumbar, coccygeal, and sacral nerves are found.

Causalgia (cawx-al-jah)

A pain condition where burning sensations develop from a peripheral nerve.

CBT

Cognitive-behavioral therapy. This is a practice that focuses on identifying new patterns of behaving and thinking that may influence a person's feelings. The concept explains how thoughts and feelings may influence the behaviors that one engages in.

Central Nervous System

Also called the CNS. This is the part of the body that includes the brain, spinal cord, and meninges that are responsible for conveying information throughout all parts of the body.

Cerebellum (sar-e-bell-um)

A segment of the brain in the posterior part of the skull behind the brainstem. The cerebellum controls voluntary muscle functions and balance.

Cerebral Contusion

A bruise in the cerebral area. The condition may develop due to fatigue, in particular from blows to the head. The issue may trigger a general inability to perform certain mental functions.

Cerebral Edema

When fluid builds up in the brain area. The condition causes the brain to swell.

Cerebral Hemorrhage

When a blood vessel in the brain breaks apart resulting in bleeding. The bleeding may develop in part of the brain or throughout the entire organ.

Cerebral Palsy

Also known as CP. A condition that causes a person's muscle tones to be impaired. This may result in an impairment of motor skills and movement. The issue develops in childhood due to brain damage.

Cerebrospinal Fluid (ser-ee-bro-spy-nul)

A fluid that is produced in the choroid plexus. The fluid moves around the brain, spinal cord, and surrounding tissues. The fluid keeps the tissues hydrated and ensures they continue to move properly.

Cerebrovascular Accident (ser-ee-bro-vas-ku-lur)

Another word for a stroke. The condition develops when the blood flow to the brain is blocked, either from a blood clot or a tumor.

Cerebrum (sur-ree-brum)

The upper part of the brain. The tissue maintains and controls voluntary body functions. This also supports intellectual functions.

Cervical Radiculopathy

A pinched nerve that develops when a nerve in the neck exits the spinal canal.

Claustrophobia (clos-troh-foe-be-ah)

Fear of tight spaces

Coma (koe-ma)

A deep form of unconsciousness where a person is not able to give motor signals. The person may still be breathing.

Concussion (kun-kush-in)

A brain injury that develops when the brain deflects off the cranium. This is noted by intense fatigue that develops in the brain.

Conditioning

A form of learning that pairs a conditioned stimulus with a separate unconditioned stimulus. The brain will establish a link between the stimuli and certain events or activities. A conditioned reflex may develop as a response to stimuli.

Delirium (de-leer-ee-um)

A condition where a person becomes confused. This may be caused by medications or from a surgical procedure, although some illnesses may also be a factor.

Delirium Tremens (tre-mins)

Also called DTs. A form of delirium that occurs when a person experiences alcohol withdrawal. This may involve sudden changes in one's heart rate and general confusion. Sweating may also accompany the issue.

Delusion

When a person believes something that is in actuality false.

Dementia (dem-en-sha)

A series of symptoms produced by a brain disorder. This may be brought on due to a stroke or a degenerative concern like Alzheimer's.

Dendrite (den-drite)

A branch that leads off a nerve cell. The dendrite will respond to a stimulus from another neuron in the system.

Diplegia (di-plee-jah)

Paralysis that involves both sides of the body.

Dopamine (doe-pah-mean)

A neurotransmitter released by nerve cells. The compound influences a person's motivations for behaviors.

Dura Mater (dur-ah may-tur)

A membrane that covers and protects the brain and spinal cord. The compound is thick and has a leathery feel to it.

Dyslexia (dis lex-ee-ah)

A concern where the brain is unable to process oral and written content properly.

Echoencephalography (ek-oh-en-cee-fal-ogra-fee)

A test that uses ultrasonic waves to identify how the brain and other functions within the skull operate.

ECT

Electroconvulsive therapy. Also called electroshock therapy. A series of electric currents move through the brain to trigger a mild seizure. The treatment helps to control brain chemistry functions and potentially reduces the intensity of some mental health concerns.

EEG

Electroencephalogram. The brain is examined with electrodes placed along the scalp. The brain's activities are analyzed to identify any possible abnormalities in the functions of the brain.

Efferent Pathways

The movement of nerve structures that transfer impulses from a nerve center to a peripheral site.

Eidetic (ey-dee-tick)

Relating to the ability of a person to properly visualize things that one notices based on prior events or experiences.

Encephalitis (en-sef-al-eye-tis)

Inflammation in the brain. Characterized by headaches, lethargy, and stiffness in the neck.

Ependyma (ep-en-dee-mah)

A membrane that lines the central canal and ventricles in the spinal column.

Epidural (ep-i-dur-ul)

Over the dura mater.

Epidural Anesthesia

Anesthesia that is applied in the epidural area.

Epilepsy (ep-ill-ep-see)

A condition where a person frequently has seizures.

Epineurium (e-pin-ur-ee-um)

The covering of a peripheral nerve.

Factitious Disorder (fack-tish-us)

The condition is also called Munchausen Syndrome A condition where a person acts as though they have a condition even though they are not actually ill.

Frontal Lobe

A segment of the cerebral hemisphere anterior to the central sulcus and lateral sulcus. The segment influences behaviors relating to behavior, learning, and voluntary movements.

Ganglion (gang-lee-in)

A structure in the peripheral nervous system that involves a series of nerve cells.

Glasgow Coma Scale

A measurement of consciousness following a traumatic brain injury. A person's ability to open the eyes, respond verbally, and to have proper motor responses is measured. The highest possible score on the scale is 15, which means a person is fully responsive and has not experienced any damages. The lowest score is a 3, which means that a person is either dead or is in a deep coma.

Guillain-Barre Syndrome

A condition where a person experiences damages to the nerves following an attack on the immune system. The condition may be preceded by a viral infection.

Hallucination (hal-oo-sin-ay-shun)

A case where a person sees things that they feel are real, but they are not. This may be related to things that one sees in the mind. This is a common condition among those with various brain conditions.

Hemorrhagic Stroke

The condition is also known as an aneurysm. A condition where a person experiences a blood vessel rupturing in the brain. This will cause a stroke.

Hippocampus (hip-oh-cam-pus)

A segment of gray matter found on the temporal lobe. The tissue helps process memory-related functions.

Hydrocephalus (high-droe-sef-al-us)

When the brain develops an excess amount of cerebrospinal fluid.

Hyperesthesia (high-pur-es-tee-sha)

When a person becomes overly sensitive to a sensory impact.

Hypnosis (hip-noe-sis)

When a person falls into a state where they are increasingly receptive to suggestions and ideas. The process is induced by another person.

Hypochondria (high-poe-kon-dree-ah)

A general fear about one's health. This includes a person believing that they will become ill or may already be ill. This is in spite of there being no evidence that they are ill.

Hypochondriasis (high-poe-kon-dree-aye-sis)

When a person is afraid of having a medical condition.

Hysteria

Excess emotion. The condition is difficult to control. In most cases, the hysteria refers to fear or panic.

Interneurons

A series of neurons that connect to each other to support certain physical activities.

Intracranial Hematoma (hee-mah-toe-mah)

Blood that builds up within the brain or in the area between the brain and skull.

Intracranial Pressure

A measure of the pressure of the cerebrospinal fluid in the brain and the brain tissue in general. The ICP is measured after an injury to identify how well the brain is responding to therapy and treatment following an injury.

Intelligence Quotient

Also referred to as IQ. A number that refers to a person's ability to use reason and to solve problems. This is in comparison with the statistical norm for one's age. The general average is 100. Those who have an IQ of 130 or higher are interpreted as being superior in intelligence. People who have an IQ of under 70 may be interpreted as being mentally impaired, although the definition may vary.

Ischemic Stroke (is-kem-ick)

A stroke that develops when a blood vessel is blocked.

Lethargy (leth-ar-gee)

A condition where a person frequently feels tired and listless.

Level of Consciousness

May be called LOC. When a person experiences a measurement of arousal or interest. This includes how a person is aroused and how they may respond to certain activities or things in their environment.

Loss of Consciousness

Occurs when a person experiences a reduction in blood flow and oxygen to the brain. The concern is often temporary, although the amount of time the person loses consciousness may vary. Also known as LOC; this is not to be confused with the level of consciousness.

Lumbar Puncture

Also referred to as a spinal tap or LP procedure. Fluid is collected from the spinal area in the lower back through a needle. The test is to identify any possible concerns that might have developed within the central nervous system.

Mental Age

A person's mental functionality based on age and is compared to the norm. For instance, a person who is younger and has an older mental age may have a mental capacity greater than others of that same physical age.

Mandibular Nerve (man-dib-u-lur)

The nerve that influences the chewing functions. This includes the ability to feel the chewing sensations and to identify when chewing is completed.

Mania

A strong sense of elation. This may also include having an obsession with something.

Median Nerve

A nerve found in the arm. The nerve triggers sensor and motor motions to the hand and arm.

Medulla Oblongata (med-oo-la ob-long-at-ah)

The lower part of the brain stem. The organ, or MO, conveys information between the brain and spinal cord. The MO will influence the functionality of cardiac and reflex functions in the body.

Megalomania (may-gah-loe-ma-nee-ah)

An obsession with wealth or power. This may include a person thinking that they are more important or powerful than others.

Meninges (men-in-gees)

Membranes that cover the brain and spinal column.

Meningioma (men-in-gee-oh-mah)

A neoplasm situated in the central nervous system. The condition may be benign, although some conditions may also be malignant.

Meningitis (men-inj-eye-tis)

An inflammation that develops in the membranes that cover the brain and spinal cord. The inflammation may be triggered by an outside bacteria or from a viral infection. Treatment is required as soon as possible to prevent possible amputations or other consequences.

Meningocele (men-in-joe-cell)

A birth defect where a sac protrudes out of the spinal column. The defect will include spinal fluid but no neural tissues. Membranes intended to cover the nervous system may cover the meningocele in spite of the tissue not having any proper function. Surgery may be performed to correct the issue.

Merkel Cells (mur-kul)

Epidermal cells in the startum basale, the inside layer of the epidermis. The cells are in an area like the fingertips where sensory information may be easier to gather.

Microcephaly (mi-crow-sef-al-ee)

A condition where the head is smaller than what it should be for one's body.

Migraine (my-grain)

A headache that is more severe than usual. The condition may cause weakness, nausea, and increased sensitivity to light and sound.

Minimal Brain Dysfunction

Also known as MBD. This is a term used to identify when a person has difficulty remembering things. The term has been mostly replaced with attention deficit disorder or attention deficit hyperactivity disorder, although MBD may still be used in some reports.

Multiple Sclerosis (sk-lur-oh-sis)

Also known as MS. The immune system destroys the protective coverings of nerves in the body, thus causing damages to how the body's nervous system cells connect with each other. As nerve impulses are disrupted, a person will become weak and fatigued. Coordination may be impaired. In other cases, a person may develop vision loss or double vision. While some people may be symptom-free for extended periods, there are also times when flare-ups may develop. Chronic symptoms that do not go away may also be a problem.

Myelin (my-lin)

A fatty material that covers axons and nerve fibers in the body. The material insulates the nerves and improves how messages are sent.

Myelitis (my-lye-tis)

Inflammation in the spinal cord.

Myelography (my-lo-gra-fee)

An examination of the spinal cord using a CT scan or x-ray to identify possible irregularities in the tissue. A contrast dye is administered to make the tissue more noticeable during the exam process.

Narcolepsy (nar-coe-lep-see)

A brain condition that involves sleep-wake cycles that are not controlled properly.

Negativism (neg-a-tiv-izm)

Behavior that indicates a person being overly skeptical of the advice of others. This includes a person being increasingly resistant to suggestions and advice.

Neocortex (nee-oh-kor-tex)

A part of the cerebral cortex that focuses on language, memory, reasoning, and thought. The neocortex also identifies sensory information transmitted from other parts of the body.

Nerve

A small structure within the body that has fibers that conduct impulses. These signals travel from the central nervous system to other parts of the body. The nerves are necessary to trigger physical functions and to identify particular activities that may develop in the body.

Nerve Block

Blockage of neural activities. This is due to an anesthetic agent being administered. The nerve block may be used during a surgical procedure as a means of keeping a patient from feeling pain.

Neural Conduction

Nerve impulses that go along a nerve and move away from a stimulus.

Nerve Growth Factor

Also known as NGF. A material that regulates growth functions and how neurons are received by the body. This may be interpreted as a growth factor in the body.

Neuralgia (newr-al-jah)

Pains that develop along a cranial nerve.

Neural Tube Defect

A birth defect that develops within the brain, spine, or spinal column. The condition develops during the first month of the pregnancy. The issue may involve the spinal column not forming properly or not closing properly. These are issues that may be noticed during the pregnancy itself through a traditional ultrasound test.

Neurapraxia (newr-a-prax-ee-ah)

Damage to the peripheral nerve. The body will temporarily lose control of its impulses.

Neurasthenia (newr-a-sten-ee-ah)

A condition where a person experiences consistent fatigue and physiologic difficulties.

Neuritis (newr-eye-tis)

Inflammation in a nerve. The condition is painful and may result in temporary paralysis.

Neurocytoma (newr-oe-sigh-toe-ma)

A brain tumor that includes cells that come from the nervous system.

Neurofibroma (newr-oe-fibe-roe-ma)

A tumor that develops from fibroblasts and other cells with nerve fibers entering the tissue. The condition is benign, although it can be firm and may cause pains in most cases.

Neurofibrosarcoma (newr-oh-fibe-ro-sar-koe-ma)

A malignant tumor in the nerves. The tumor develops from cutaneous nerves in the body and may spread into other tissues through metastasis.

Neurogenesis (newr-oe-gen-eh-sis)

The creation of neurons where stem cells divide so that various cells become neurons. The process assists in the production of healthy nerve connections and brain functionality.

Neuroglia (newr-aw-glee-ah)

Tissues that support the development of the nervous system.

Neurological (newr-owe-lodge-ick-ul)

Relating to the nervous system.

Neuroma (newr-owe-mah)

A neoplasm that develops in the body. The benign condition involves nerve cells and fibers.

Neuron (newr-on)

A cellular unit of nervous tissue. The neuron is a body and an axon that supports the impulses in the nervous system. Dendrites are included to help move information between neurons and to conduct physical activities while triggering sensations.

Neuroretinitis (newr-oe-ret-in-eye-tis)

Inflammation in the optic nerve and the retina.

Neurotransmitter (newr-oe-trans-mit-tur)

A chemical compound that conveys messages to other cells in the body.

Neurotropic (newr-oe-trop-ick)

Growing new neural tissues.

Obsessive-Compulsive Disorder

Also called OCD. A disorder where a person experiences frequent thoughts or obsessions along with regular behaviors or compulsions. These are actions that a person has and is a regular desire to repeat some action many times over. The symptoms may gradually form and can influence one's daily life.

Obtund

An effort to weaken the pains that a person feels.

Oculomotor Nerve (ock-ue-lo-mo-ter)

A nerve that goes through the cavernous sinus and out through the skull into the orbit. The nerve assists in supporting the sensory information felt in the eye and orbit.

Olfactory Nerve (ol-fack-tur-ee)

A cranial nerve that transmits the body's sense of smell. This is the first of the ten cranial nerves that originate from the skull.

Optic Nerve

The second of the cranial nerves. The nerve transfers visual information to the brain.

Panic

A sensation where a person develops intense fear and anxiety. The feeling may develop from something irrational.

Panic Attack

A response to fear that is intense in comparison with the situation.

Paranoia

A feeling where someone is overly suspicious about someone or something. This is a concern that may include irrational thoughts or feelings about others. The condition is not always reflective of a paranoid personality disorder or schizophrenia. In some cases, a person may feel paranoia and may still think clearly. However, that person might have an emotional response that resembles a state of delusion.

Paresthesia

A condition where the skin feels numb or starts tingling. The condition starts to develop without any known causes.

Parietal Lobe

The top central part of the cerebral hemisphere. The area is located near the central sulcus and occipital lobe.

Parkinson Disease

Also known as PD. A disease that influences movement. The condition develops in the nervous system and damages neurons responsible for supporting regular movements in the body. The condition may trigger shaking and other physical functions that are not easily controlled. Some hallucinations may also develop due to the issue.

Peripheral Neuropathy

Damages to the peripheral nerves that keep movements and sensations from operating properly. Organ functions may also be impaired in the most significant cases.

Phantom Limb

A condition where a person feels sensations in an area where a limb is absent. This is common among those who have had amputations of part of or an entire limb.

PNS

Peripheral nervous system. The system involves the autonomic functions in the body including promoting healthy muscle functions. The PNS includes the nerves that are outside of the brain and spinal cord.

Polyneuropathy (pol-e-newr-op-ath-ee)

A condition where many peripheral nerves are simultaneously impacted.

Pons (ponz)

The front area of the hindbrain. The region is between the medulla and midbrain. The pons supports the transmission of nerve signals between neural pathways.

Prosencephalon (pro-sen-sef-al-on)

The front part of the brain.

PTSD

Post-traumatic stress disorder. The concern occurs among people who have experienced traumatic events in the past. This may include an elevated risk of concern over a certain activity or the fear that something may develop. The concern can be marked by some feelings of aversion to certain things that might relate to what someone is afraid of.

Pudendal Nerve (pu-den-dul)

A nerve that develops in the sacral spinal cord. The nerve influences the genitalia, sphincter, and urethral sphincter. The condition may be damaged in childbirth.

Radial Nerve

A nerve located along the upper arm. The nerve starts in the upper thoracic spinal cord and attaches to the posterior cord. The nerve triggers functionality in the arm and extension.

Radiculopathy (ra-dik-u-lo-path-ee)

A pinched nerve. A nerve will not work properly resulting in pains and weakness in an area. The root of the nerve is impacted the most.

Reflex

A sudden movement that develops as a stimulus to an event that occurs. This may include a stimulus surrounding activities that are transmitted to the brain or spinal cord. The reflex is usually involuntary.

Reflex Arc

How a reflex is formed and how the movement may change.

REM

Rapid eye movement. This is the fast motion of a person's eyes during sleep. This is a stage when a person attains a condition where the eyes move quickly while sleeping. The patient may experience vivid dreams at this point.

Reye's Syndrome (rayz)

A condition that appears as swelling in the brain and liver. This may develop in those who have experienced the flu or varicella infection. The condition is elevated in children who take aspirin. Those who are sensitive to aspirin are at a high risk of the issue if they consume the drug.

RIND

Reversible ischemic neurologic deficit. The effects that may come from an ischemic attack.

Seasonal Affective Disorder

Also known as SAD or seasonal depression. A person may develop depression at a certain time in the year. The condition develops mainly in the fall and winter months in most cases. The concern may be treated through light therapy.

Schizophrenia (skit-zo-fren-ee-ah)

A mental disorder where a person is unable to think and act clearly. This includes a person feeling as though they are no longer in control of their reality. The issue may cause concentration issues and cases where a person experiences things that are not actually happening. A person may also experience an inability to interact with others normally or safely.

Sciatic Nerve (sigh-at-ick)

A nerve that develops in the lumbar and sacral spinal cord. The nerve triggers motor and sensory functions in the lower part of the body. This nerve is the largest one in the body.

Sciatica (sigh-at-ick-ah)

Pain in the sciatic nerve. The sensations will develop in the lower back and move down to the leg.

Seizure (see-sure)

A surge in the electrical functions in the brain. The condition will impact movements and awareness for a brief time. The condition may also trigger pains in the head. The condition may last for a few seconds, although some people may develop seizures that take place several times a day.

Spinal Cord

The part of the central nervous system that is secured in the vertebral column.

Spinal Nerve

A nerve that forms in the spinal column through the dorsal and ventral spinal roots. There are 31 of these nerves in the body with each working for different segments in the spinal cord.

Spinal Puncture

A process where fluid is collected from between the third and fourth lumbar vertebrae. The test on the fluid identifies if there are concerns in the spinal fluid and if there is a possible infection.

Spinal Stenosis (sten-oh-sis)

When the spinal canal becomes narrow.

Superego

A part of the personality that focuses on ethics and standards. This includes considering self-analysis.

Sural Nerve (sur-ul)

A part of the tibial nerve that will send sensory information to parts of the lower leg and foot.

Synapse (sin-apps)

An area located in between two nerves or between a nerve and an organ that may be impacted.

Tectospinal (teck-toe-spy-nul)

Relating to nerve fibers that will are found from the mesencephalic tectum to the spinal cord.

Telencephalon (tell-en-sef-al-on)

The division of the front part of the brain that will produce the olfactory bulbs, basal ganglia, and cerebral cortex.

Temporal Lobe

A division of the brain that produces the auditory and semantic functions in the body.

TENS

Transcutaneous electrical nerve stimulation. The practice uses a series of electrodes linked to the brain or other nerves in the body. The practice helps restore the functionality of nerves in the body. This includes helping those nerves become fully restored or to possibly relieve pains that may develop due to nerve-related disorders.

Terminal Nerve

The nerve that appears at the main part of the skull. This is where the cranial nerves end.

Tetanus (tet-nus)

Also known as lockjaw. An infection that impacts the central nervous system due to the Clostridium tetani toxin. The protein may enter the body through a laceration or puncture wound. The condition can cause muscle spasms and paralysis and may lead to death in some cases unless the issue is treated.

Thalamus (thal-a-mus)

A segment in the brain that includes mostly gray matter. The tissue transfers sensory information throughout the body and also influences how well the body can identify pains.

Thermoalgesia (thur-moe-al-geez-ee-ah)

Pains that may develop when a part of the body feels warm.

Transient Ischemic Attack

Also known as TIA or a mini-stroke. The stroke lasts for a few minutes on average. Blood flow to the brain will be blocked for a brief time. The condition will cause numbness or weakness in the body and will most often influence one side of the body. The condition requires immediate medical attention to ensure that it can be distinguished from an actual stroke.

Titubation (tit-ue-bay-shun)

When a person is walking with a noticeable gait. This may be a sign that a person may stumble and struggle with walking normally.

Tourette's Syndrome (tour-etz)

A disorder where a person experiences various vocal and motor tics many times in a day. The concern may develop over an extensive period. The tics are not easily controlled.

Tractotomy (track-tot-oe-mee)

A surgical treatment where a nerve tract receives an incision. The treatment helps to relieve pains.

Trance (trans-e)

A state of consciousness where a person appears to be asleep but is slightly aware of their surroundings. The condition may cause a person's motor functions to become weakened.

Tranquilizer (tran-quill-eye-zur)

A drug that will reduce stress in the body while maintaining a natural mental functionality.

Transference (trans-fur-ince)

A case where a person transfers feelings that were associated in their early life. The feelings might be applied to occasions or interaction with other people to change a mood or attitude. The activity is unconscious behavior.

Trichotillomania (trick-oh-til-oh-main-ee-ah)

A mental concern where a person frequently has a desire to pull their own hair.

Trigeminal (trig-em-in-ul)

Relating to the fifth cranial nerve. The nerve involves the face and various motor functions of the face. This is the largest cranial nerve.

Trigeminal Neuralgia (try-gem-in-ul nur-al-jah)

Inflammation in the trigeminal nerve. The inflammation may cause intense pains and spams around the face.

Unconsciousness

A case where a person loses awareness of their surroundings. This includes a person being unable to respond to sensory stimuli. The condition may be temporary, but a prolonged period suggests that a person may be in a coma.

Vagus Nerve (vay-gus)

The tenth cranial nerve. The nerve influences the heart, lungs, and digestive tract.

White Matter

The part of the central nervous system that has a lighter appearance when compared with other areas. The area is informally referred to as gray matter. The area includes nerve fibers and some neuronal cell bodies and dendrites. The area allows messages to be transferred between one area and another.

Vestibule (ves-ti-bule)

An opening or channel that moves into another area. This may include one channel that forms in the nervous system and leads to another segment in the area.

Prefixes

astr/o	star
atelo	incomplete
caus/o	burning sensation
cerebell/o	cerebellum
cerebr/o	cerebrum
concuss/o	shaking together
contus/o	bruise
dolor/o	pain
dur/o	dura matter, or something hard
encephal/o	brain
esthes/o	nerve sensations or feelings
ganglion/o	ganglion
gli/o	feeling like glue
gnos/o	sense of knowledge
hedon/o	pleasure
hypn/o	pertaining to sleep
kelpt/o	to steal
log	speech

logo	words
mening/o	membranes
ment/o	mind
myel/o	spinal cord
narc/o	sleep or feeling numb
neuri	nervous system
odyn	pain
phob/o	fear or a desire to avoid
piez/o	pressure
psych/o	mind
radicul/o	nerve root
rhiz/o	root
schiz	division
somn/o	sleep
synaps/o	point of contact or synapse
syring/o	tube or pipe that may be inserted in the body
taut	similar
vag/o	vagus nerve
vestibul/o	vestibule

Chapter 9 – Reproductive System

The reproductive system refers to all the parts of the body necessary for sexual reproduction and functionality. Part of this includes the hormones and pheromones that are necessary for the reproductive system to stay healthy.

The terms in this chapter include important details about pregnancies. This includes recognizing how a woman's body evolves and changes during her pregnancy. Considerations surrounding the abortion process or any other procedure that may take place due to concerns about pregnancy are also covered.

Abortifacient (ah-bore-tif-ay-shint)

A medication that triggers the abortive process.

Acrosome (ack-roe-so-muh)

A material that covers the anterior part of the spermatozoon. The area contains the enzymes that are required to allow the sperm to penetrate the egg.

Adrenarche (ad-ren-ark)

A process that develops in a child's body at around seven to eight years of age when the child's adrenal glands start to mature. This leads to the elevated production of androstenedione as well as other androgens. The process continues during puberty.

AFP

Alpha-fetoprotein. This is a protein generated in the liver of the developing fetus. The AFP may move through the placenta and eventually into the mother's blood. A test may be conducted to identify the AFP levels of the woman's blood during the second trimester.

Afterbirth

The materials that are cleared from the uterus following the birthing process. This includes the placenta and umbilical cord among other membranes in the uterus.

Amenorrhea (a-men-or-he-ah)

A condition when the woman is not menstruating. This may be a sign of an eating disorder or a blockage in the body.

Ammion (am-ee-in)

A sac found around the embryo.

Amniocentesis (am-nee-oh-sen-tee-sis)

A test used to identify possible infections in the unborn child. This includes possible chromosomal mutations. The test requires fluid to be removed from the amniotic sac to determine the condition.

Amniotic Fluid (am-nee-aw-tik)

A clear fluid that surrounds the fetus during its development. The fluid allows the fetus to remain suspended to ensure it will not be at risk of injury.

Androgen (an-droe-gin)

Steroidal hormone that enhances the development of the male organs. The androgen triggers the development of muscles. This may also lead to hair growth and changes in one's voice.

Andropause (an-droe-paws)

Male menopause, or a concern where the man is not getting the androgens that he requires.

Androsterone (an-droe-stare-own)

A compound that is based on testosterone or androstenedione. The compound may be found in some medications used to restore the body's functions.

Anovulation (an-oh-vue-lay-shun)

When the ovaries no longer ovulate.

Antepartal Care (an-tay-par-tal)

Health care that may be provided to a woman during or after a pregnancy.

Apgar Score (ap-gar)

An assessment to identify the health of a newborn baby. The score is determined based on the skin color, the child's pulse, physical activity, facial expressions, and respiration. Each point is based on a score from 0 to 2. A higher score suggests that the child is healthy and does not require any added care following its birth.

Aphrodisiac (af-roe-dee-see-ack)

A compound that triggers sexual activities and interests.

Aplasia (ap-lay-sha)

The improper development of an organ or tissue in the body.

Areola (air-ee-oh-la)

A ring of skin that surrounds the nipple. The skin appears pigmented and may be slightly raised from the rest of the area.

ASC-US

Atypical squamous cells of undetermined significance. These may be found in a Pap test and can be used in cases where the doctor is uncertain about the quality of certain cervical cells. The cells may be cancerous or precancerous, or they may not be signs of any potential cancer developments at all.

Aspermia (as-pur-mee-ah)

An issue where the body is not producing semen.

Ateliosis (ae-te-lee-oh-sis)

A form of dwarfism. This includes the body not being fully sexually matured.

Azoospermia (ae-zoo-spur-mee-ah)

A lack of sperm in the male ejaculate.

Balanitis (bal-an-eye-tis)

Inflammation of the penis tip and foreskin.

Balanoposthitis (bal-an-oh-post-high-tis)

Inflammation in the uncircumcised penis.

Benign Prostatic Hyperplasia (high-per-play-shah)

Also known as BPH. The condition occurs as the prostate becomes enlarged and presses its way into other tissues. Older persons are more likely to develop the condition. The issue causes a person to have a need to urine more often. The issue may become worse at night. Although the condition is benign, this may be interpreted as a precursor to prostate cancer.

Bisexuality

A case where a person develops a sexual attraction to people of both sexes.

Breast

The mammary gland in the female body, although this may develop in a man depending on how hormonal functions develop.

Breastfeeding

A process where a woman feeds a baby through the breast tissue. Breast milk is given to the baby. This is not done by all mothers, although it may help enhance the bond between the child and the mother.

BSE

Breast self-exam. The process is recommended for all women to help them identify any possible growths or other concerns that may suggest breast cancer.

Castration (kass-tray-shun)

A process where the sex gland is removed.

Caul (call)

A sac that includes amniotic fluid. The sac covers the fetus.

Cervical Dysplasia (dis-play-sha)

The development of cells on the outside surface of the cervix. The concern may be unusual in nature and could be a sign of possible cancer development.

Cervicitis (ser-vik-eye-tis)

Inflammation in the cervix.

Cervix (ser-vix)

A section in the uterus that is located between the vagina and lower isthmus. The area is shaped like a canal and is necessary for the birthing process.

Cesarean Section (ses-air-ee-in)

A surgical procedure where a person delivers a fetus through the abdominal wall and uterus. The process is used in cases where the natural birthing process cannot possibly be done without risking the life of the mother or the child.

Chlamydia (kla-mid-dee-ah)

A bacterial infection that can be transmitted sexually. The condition can result in painful urination, although not all people will experience symptoms from the condition.

Chordoma (kor-doh-ma)

A malignant tumor that is produced from the embryonic materials in the notochord.

Chorion (kore-ee-on)

An embryonic membrane that goes over the embryo. This is the outside sac to protect the unborn child. The chorion will develop into the production of the placenta.

Chorionic Villus Sampling (kor-ee-on-ik vil-us)

A test that identifies possible chromosome-related issues. A tissue sample is collected from the chorion to identify any possible concerns in the body.

Circumcision (sur-cum-sih-shun)

A process where the foreskin on the penis is removed. This requires a surgical cut.

Clitoris (klit-or-iss)

A structure that is found in the female body along the far ends of the labia minora. For men, the structure is in the penis and supports erectile functions under the labial commissure.

Coitus (koi-tus)

A technical term for sexual intercourse.

Colostrum (kol-os-trum)

Breast milk that the mother produces late in her pregnancy. The milk has a higher antibody and protein content. It is recommended that the mother's milk is pumped at this time and then provided to the child during the first days of life.

Colposcopy (kolp-os-caw-pee)

A review of the vagina and cervix through an endoscope. The endoscope is inserted into the vagina.

Colpotomy (kolp-ot-oe-mee)

An incision procedure in the vaginal area for a surgical procedure.

Conception

The time when the sperm enters the ova. This is when pregnancy officially begins.

Condom

A material that is applied over the penis during sex to ensure the pregnancy is prevented or a sexually transmitted disease is not be transferred. A female condom may also be applied over the cervical and vaginal tissue, although a condom is more associated with male use.

Consanguinity (con-sang-win-i-tee)

The relationship that people have with one another. This refers to people having the same ancestor. The consideration may be a predictor in determining if certain people might have particular conditions.

Contraception

A practice designed to prevent pregnancy or the transmission of a sexually transmitted disease. It requires the parties involved to apply the appropriate materials over their sexual organs before engaging in sexual activities.

Contraction

A case where the tension produced becomes intense. This is related mostly to pregnancy as it involves added tension in the birth canal. The uterus will become tight and will do so rhythmically with the contractions coming at intervals.

Copulation

A general sexual link between two people.

Dilation and Curettage

Also known as D&C. The process involves tissue being removed from the uterus. This is to treat heavy bleeding conditions, although it may also be used to eliminate the lining of the uterus after an abortion or miscarriage.

Decidua (de-sid-ue-ah)

A membrane that is found in the lining of the wall in the uterus. The decidua is formed during the pregnancy.

Dysfunctional Uterine Bleeding

A concern where a woman experiences vaginal bleeding beyond the regular menstrual cycle. The issue may be triggered by hormonal issues or from the use of some medications.

Dysmenorrhea (dis-men-or-hee-ah)

Cramps that develop before or during a menstrual period.

Dystocia (dis-toe-see-ah)

Difficulty with the child birthing process. This may include intense distress that may put the life of the mother or the child at risk.

Eclampsia (ee-clamp-see-ah)

A condition where seizures develop following the woman's pregnancy. This may occur when the blood pressure level is too high or there is a large amount of protein in her urine. The condition may trigger intense convulsions and could result in a coma in some cases. The concern may also be worse if any organs are being impacted during the pregnancy.

Ectopic Pregnancy (e-top-ik)

A condition where a fertilized egg develops outside of the uterus. A surgical procedure is required to remove the egg as the unborn child will not survive outside of the uterus.

Egg

A reproductive cell in the female body. The egg needs to be fertilized by the sperm to trigger pregnancy.

Ejaculation (ee-jack-ue-lay-shun)

The removal of semen from the male urethra. This occurs suddenly and often develops following an erection, although it may also be triggered by sexual activities.

Embryo (em-bree-oh)

The earliest form of an organism. This is when the organism is ready to develop into a larger body.

Endocervicitis (en-doe-sur-vi-sigh-tis)

Inflammation in the mucus along the uterine cervix.

Endoderm (en-doe-durm)

The inside part of the three layers in an embryo.

Endometrium (en-doe-mee-tree-um)

A mucous membrane that surrounds the uterus.

Endometriosis (en-doe-me-tree-oh-sis)

A condition where tissue that regularly grows inside the uterus starts to grow outside the uterus. The concern can develop anywhere in the abdominal cavity. The concern may also trigger intense pains in the body.

Epididymis (ep-id-id-ee-mis)

A structure found within the scrotum. This is a cord-shaped organ that connects to the back part of the testes. The area secures the sperm.

Epididymitis (ep-eh-did-e-my-tis)

Inflammation in the epididymis.

Episiotomy (ep-eez-ee-ot-toe-mee)

A surgical cut in the perineum. The cut widens the vaginal opening to facilitate an easier childbirth.

Erectile Dysfunction

Also known as ED or impotence. A case where a man is unable to develop an erection. This is an age-related concern, although it may be caused by injuries to the penile area or from nerves no longer functioning as well in the region.

Estimated Date of Delivery

The time in the pregnancy when a mother is expected to give birth. This is referenced as the EDD in an official report. The timeframe may be determined based on how the mother's pregnancy is progressing or calculated from the approximate time when the conception might have taken place.

Fallopian Tubes (fal-oh-pee-in)

A pair of muscle canals in the female body. The canals allow the ovum to move from the ovary to the uterus.

Fetal (fee-tul)

Relating to the fetus.

Fetal Heart Rate

A measure of the heart rate of the fetus during the pregnancy. The rate should be measured at varying times during the pregnancy. The ideal FHR should be 120 to 160 beats per minute (bpm) during the earliest stages of the pregnancy and then around 170 bpm at ten weeks. The FHR should be around 130 bpm during birth.

Fetus (fee-tis)

An embryo of a being during the late parts of its development.

Fibroadenoma (fy-bro-ad-een-oe-ma)

Benign tumors that form in the breast tissues. These are not expected to influence the woman's risk of developing breast cancer in the future. The growths may include some oval shapes and some slight rubbery feelings. These tumors do not cause pains.

Fibrocystic Breast Disease

A benign disease where the breast develops a slightly lumpy appearance. The breasts feel sore and the woman may experience some pains, which may be worse during a period. The condition is not expected to influence the risk of developing breast cancer.

FTND

Full-term normal delivery. This occurs when a child is delivered properly and normally.

FTT

Failure to thrive. The child may not have gained enough weight or might have lost more weight than normal. This is a concern that may develop after a child's birth and must be monitored carefully.

Galactorrhea (gal-ack-taur-e-ah)

Excess lactation

Galactose (gal-ack-tose)

A sugar found in lactose, a protein included in milk. The mother's milk can be tested to identify how well the body is producing sugar.

Gamete (gam-eat)

A sex cell that has matured.

GDM

Gestational diabetes mellitus. A concern where a woman develops diabetes during pregnancy. This may be caused by the body not being capable to tolerate glucose correctly. The concern may also be caused by placental hormones that trigger blood sugar spikes. The diabetes issue should be relieved after the pregnancy ends, although the woman may be at a higher risk of Type II diabetes later in her life.

Gene

A compound in the human body that carries a particular trait on a chromosome. The compound will influence how the body responds to certain functions.

Genetic

Relating to reproductive activities or from a person's birth.

Genitalia

Referring to the sexual or reproductive organs.

Gestation (jes-tay-shun)

The period from fertilization to birth.

Gonad (goe-nad)

A sex gland. This refers to the ovaries or testes.

Gonadal (goe-nad-ul)

Relating to a gonad.

Gonorrhea (gone-or-ree-ah)

A sexually transmitted disease. The bacterial issue may cause infertility if not treated. The concern may also cause pains when urinating or an unusual discharge coming from the genital area.

Gravida (grav-id-ah)

A reference to pregnancy. This refers to the number of pregnancies that a woman has had. This is regardless of whether or not the pregnancy was successful and was carried to full term.

Gravidity

A reference to when a woman is pregnant.

Gynecology

Relating to the treatment of conditions relating to women. This particularly focuses on breast and genital-related concerns that a woman might have.

Hematocolpos (he-mah-toe-coal-pus)

Excessive development of menstrual blood in the vaginal tissue.

Hematometra (he-mah-toe-met-ra)

The development of excess menstrual blood in the uterus.

Hematospermia (hem-ah-toe-sperm-ee-ah)

Blood found in the semen.

Hemospermia (he-moe-sperm-ee-ah)

The prostate has developed inflammation or the seminal vesicles have become weak. This is a concern relating to blood in the semen.

Heredity

A medical condition has been transferred from a parent to the child. This can be noticed in the genes that a child has been given by the parent.

Herpes Simplex Virus (hur-peez)

A virus that is sexually transmitted. The condition can cause the development of sores around the mouth or genitals. The condition is also called HSV and may be divided into HSV-1 and HSV-2. HSV-1 refers to oral herpes, and HSV-2 is genital herpes. The sores can be painful and may be transferred to others.

Heterosexuality

When two people of the opposite sex are sexually attracted to one another.

Heterosis (het-ur-oh-sis)

When the offspring of two parents appear to have qualities that are greater than that of what both parents exhibit.

HGSIL

High-grade squamous intraepithelial lesion. This is a concern that may be found in a Pap test. The lesion suggests that there are precancerous cells in the cervix but not cancerous ones. The condition needs to be treated as it may lead to cancerous concerns in the body. May also be listed in a report as HSIL.

Homosexuality

When two people of the same sex develop a sexual relationship or attraction to one another.

Hormone Replacement Therapy

Also called HRT. A process where hormones are administered to the body to control the development of certain physical symptoms. The therapy is given mainly to women who are experiencing menopause.

Hydrocele (high-droe-cell)

When fluid builds up around the testicle. The concern is common among infants, although the issue should resolve itself over time.

Hymen (high-min)

A buildup of mucous membranes around the opening of the vaginal region.

Hypogonadism (high-poe-goe-nad-izm)

Low activities in the gonads. The condition leads to improper growth and a lack of sexual development.

Hypomenorrhea (high-poe-men-or-ee-ah)

A light menstrual blood flow.

Hysterectomy (his-ter-eck-tom-ee)

The removal of the uterus through surgery. The treatment is to resolve cancerous conditions or other threats, although the procedure would cause the woman to no longer be able to become pregnant.

Hysterosalpingography (his-ter-oh-sal-ping-og-ra-fee)

An exam of the uterus and fallopian tubes. A contrast agent may be added in the tissue to help identify the tubes through an external review. Sound waves are used to identify functions in the body and to detect possible concerns that might develop in the tissues.

Hysteroscopy (his-ter-osk-op-ee)

An examination of the uterus with an endoscope placed into the vaginal area. The test visually identifies any concerns in the cavity.

Hysterotomy (his-ter-ot-om-ee)

An incision made in the uterus. The incision may be made through the vaginal area or the abdomen. The process is to facilitate a safe birthing process in complicated pregnancies, although the incision may impair future pregnancies depending on how the body responds.

IDM

Infant of diabetic mother. The child will have to be monitored and tested to identify if the child has contracted diabetes.

Impotence

A case where a man is unable to attain an erection in the penile area.

In Vitro (vee-troe)

Outside of a body. This refers to when something is produced in an environment outside of an organism. The process refers mainly to when a woman is implanted with an outside ovulation treatment if she is unable to become naturally fertilized. The process may have some risks but is the only option available in cases where a woman cannot naturally conceive.

Induction

Causing something to happen. This refers to when labor has to be induced to facilitate the healthy delivery of a baby.

Infertility

A concern where a person is unable to conceive. The issue may occur when a person being unable to produce the sperm needed for the conception process.

Inguinal Canal (in-gwin-ul)

A tunnel found in the abdominal wall. The testis will move into the scrotum.

Insemination (in-sem-in-ay-shun)

When seminal fluid is added into the vaginal area.

Intrauterine (in-tra-ute-er-in)

Inside the uterine cavity.

IUCD

Intrauterine contraceptive device. This is a T-shaped plastic device that is inserted into the uterus. It is to assist in preventing pregnancies from developing and may work for years after it is implanted. The material may also be used as an emergency form of birth control if inserted five days before having unplanned sex, although a doctor should be consulted to determine the options.

IUFD

Intrauterine fetal distress. The baby will not have received enough oxygen while in utero. This may develop during the third trimester of the pregnancy. This could cause a drop in the child's fetal heart rate, thus producing significant threats.

IUP

Intrauterine pregnancy. This is a description of the pregnancy during the first trimester. The baby can be noticed in the uterus and suggests that the pregnancy is starting normally and should be safe.

L&D

Labor and delivery, a reference to the birthing process.

Labor

A practice where the child is birthed.

Lactation

The development of milk in the mother's mammary glands.

Leiomyoma (ley-oh-my-oh-ma)

A growth found in the uterus. The issue is benign and may be found in the smooth muscle tissue. This can also be called a fibroid tumor.

Leukorrhea (lou-kor-e-ah)

Vaginal discharge during pregnancy. This is a normal event. The discharge will have a thin and white look and may produce a slight odor.

Libido (le-bee-doe)

The development of sexual interest or a desire for sex.

Low Birth Weight

When a child is born at less than 5 pounds and 8 ounces in weight. The term may be listed in a report as LBW.

LMP

Last menstrual period. This may be measured based on a woman's reporting and could be influential in determining if a woman could be pregnant. Further testing is required if it has been some time since the last period.

Lochia (loe-chee-ah)

A vaginal discharge that develops not long after childbirth. The compound includes some mucus and uterine tissue mixed with blood. This may develop up to about six weeks after birth.

Mammary Gland (mam-ur-ee)

A gland that produces milk.

Mammoplasty (mam-oh-plas-tee)

Plastic surgery on the breasts. This may involve accentuating smaller breasts or reducing the size of breasts that are too large.

Mastalgia (mas-tal-gee-ah)

Pains in the breast.

Mastopexy (mas-top-ex-ee)

Breast-lift surgery.

Menarche (men-ark)

A woman's first menstrual period.

Menopause (men-oh-paws)

When menstruation stops. This may be a concern when a woman is unable to get the proper hormones that she requires for normal functioning.

Menorrhagia (men-or-ha-gee-ah)

Excess bleeding during menstruation.

Menses (men-sis)

Blood that is discharged from the uterus during a period. The issue may include some tissues from within the body.

Menstrual Cycle

A process where a woman starts bleeding from the uterus. This may be caused by changes in how the hypothalamus and pituitary glands operate, especially as these will produce intense changes in how hormones are produced. The ovaries and genital area may also experience some changes during the cycle.

Menstruation

The general process where blood and some tissues are eliminated from the uterus. The process occurs about once a month on average. The process develops in non-pregnant women and will start in puberty and end in menopause.

Metritis (met-rye-tis)

Inflammation in the uterus.

Metrorrhagia (met-ror-hay-gee-ah)

Uterine bleeding that is unusual and is not related to the menstrual cycle.

Midwife

A person who assists a woman during the birthing process.

Miscarriage

An occasion where a fetus is lost prior to the twentieth week of pregnancy. The fetus will have died and is no longer be capable of surviving. The woman might have to undergo a surgical procedure to remove the tissue from the body.

Monorchism (mon-ork-izim)

When one testis is missing.

Morula (mor-ue-lah)

An embryo with a detailed mass.

Myometrium (my-oh-mee-tree-um)

A smooth muscle that covers the uterus.

Natal (nay-tul)

Relating to the birthing process.

Neonatal (ne-oh-nay-tul)

Relating to a new baby, or within 28 days after birth.

Neonate (ne-oh-nate)

An infant under one month of age.

Nulligravida (null-eh-grah-vee-dah)

A woman who has never been pregnant.

Nullipara (null-e-par-ah)

A woman who has never given birth. This includes a woman who has been pregnant but that event did not come to term.

Obstetrics

A field of medical study relating to the care of women who are giving birth.

Oligohydramnios (ol-eggo-high-dram-nee-ose)

A concern where the uterus has low amniotic fluid.

Oligomenorrhea (ol-geeo-men-or-hee-ah)

Light menstrual period or periods that are not happening frequently.

Oligospermia (ol-eh-goe-sper-mee-a)

When the male body is unable to develop the sperm required for regular production. This may be when a man has less than 20 million sperm for every milliliter of semen when tested.

Ontogeny (on-toe-gen-ee)

A review of the history of how well the body can develop. This includes a review of the body from its conception to maturity.

Oophorectomy (oo-for-ek-toe-mee)

When an ovary or ovaries are removed. The process is to help control cancerous developments or other threats.

Oophoritis (oo-for-eye-tis)

Inflammation in the ovary.

Orchidalgia (or-kid-al-jah)

Pains in the testicles.

Orchidectomy (or-kid-eck-toe-mee)

Removal of one or both testicles, primarily to control cancer issues.

Orchiopexy (or-kid-ee-oh-pex-ee)

Surgery to move a testicle that has not descended into the scrotum. The condition relieves any pains that may develop due to the testicle not moving all the way into the desired area.

Orchitis (ork-eye-tis)

Inflammation in one or both of the testes.

Orgasm (or-gaz-im)

The climax of sexual activity.

Ovarian Cysts

Cysts that develop in the ovary.

Ovarian Neoplasms

Tumors in the ovary. These may be cancerous or malignant, and some may be benign.

Ovary (oh-var-e)

One of the two sex glands found in the female body. The ovaries will produce hormones and ova.

Ovulation

Discharge that comes from the ovum. The discharge develops from a follicle in the ovary that has been ruptured.

Ovum (oe-vum)

A germ cell that is produced by the ovary during the ovulation process.

Pap Test

Also known as a pap smear. The test collects cells from the cervix to test them to identify evidence that cervical cancer that might have developed.

Paraphimosis (pear-a-fim-oe-sis)

A condition where the foreskin is retracted on the penile tissue but the tissue has not moved back to its original state. The condition may impair the flow of blood into the penile area and eventually cause swelling.

Parity (pear-it-e)

The number of offspring that has been produced by a woman.

Parturition (par-tur-i-shun)

The process of a woman giving birth to offspring.

Penis (pee-nis)

The male reproductive organ.

Perimenopause (pear-eh-men-oh-paws)

The time period before menopause.

Perimetritis (pear-eh-met-ree-tis)

Inflammation in the peritoneal covering in the uterus.

Perinatal (pear-e-nay-tul)

Relating to the time period immediately before and after birth. The period extends from three months before the birth to one month after birth.

Perineum (pear-in-ee-um)

The surface region between the pubic symphysis and the coccyx. This is an area found in both the male and female bodies.

Peripartum Period (per-e-par-tum)

The period right before and after the childbirth process. A woman should be carefully monitored to ensure she is capable of giving birth.

Peyronie Disease (pey-ron-ee)

A concern where plaques start to form under the penile skin. The penis will develop an unusual bending shape. The concern may make it harder for the man to develop an erection.

Phimosis (fim-oe-sis)

A concern where the foreskin is tightened or narrow. The skin cannot be retracted back to properly reveal the glans penis. This may make it difficult to urinate or to produce an erection.

PID

Pelvic inflammatory disease. An infection that causes the fallopian tubes to swell and form scar tissue to develop in the area. This may result in an infection deep within the uterine area. Pelvic pain and fatigue may develop. The concern is often triggered by sexually transmitted diseases.

PIH

Pregnancy-induced hypertension. The woman's blood pressure increases when she is pregnant. The concern may be relieved after pregnancy, although the concern may be an indicator the woman may develop hypertension later in life.

Placenta (plah-sen-tah)

An organ that develops in the uterus during pregnancy. The tissue is found along the uterine wall and will partially cover the fetus. The placenta will produce a series of hormones required to support a healthy pregnancy.

Placenta Previa (pre-vee-ah)

A concern where the placenta covers much of the cervix during the last few months of the pregnancy. The issue may require the unborn child to be repositioned to support a healthier delivery process.

PMS

Premenstrual syndrome. The condition develops in between ovulation and the period due to hormonal changes in the body. The concern can trigger fatigue and bloating in the female body and may also lead to irritability in some cases.

Polycystic Ovary Syndrome

A condition where the sex hormones in the female body are not in control. This includes estrogen and progesterone not being produced properly. The issue may result in infertility for some women.

Posset (pos-sit)

A small amount of milk that an infant may regurgitate after feeding.

Postmenopause

A period after menopause that involves emotional changes.

Postpartum

A period that develops after the woman gives birth.

Preeclampsia (pre-eh-clamp-see-ah)

A concern when a pregnant woman develops hypertension and a high amount of protein in the urine. Edema may also develop in the extremities.

Pregnancy

When a woman carries the embryo or fetus, which is the offspring, in her body before birth. The process is in utero where the development occurs.

Premature Ejaculation

An event where semen or other fluids are produced prior to sexual intercourse. This may develop prior to penetration or afterward. The concern involves the body not performing normally.

Premenopause (pre-men-oe-paws)

A period of time prior to menopause. This is when the woman has reached sexual maturity and will no longer experience regular menstrual cycles. The period may begin in one's late thirties, but it could also happen in the early fifties.

Prepuce (pre-puse)

A fold of skin that appears over the end part of the penis.

Priapism (pri-ahp-izm)

A concern where a man develops an erection that lasts for longer than average. An erection that lasts for at least four hours may result in damages to the tissues.

Primigravida (pree-mee-grah-vee-da)

A woman who has become pregnant for the first time.

Primipara (pree-mee-pear-ah)

A woman who has given birth to one child.

Prolactin (pro-lack-tin)

A hormone produced by the pituitary gland. The hormone triggers lactation in the postpartum process. A woman should have more of this hormone in her body following the birthing process, thus improving how she can nurse her child.

Prostate (pros-tait)

A male gland found under the bladder. The organ carries sperm during the ejaculation process. The gland may be found around the urethra. The organ will enlarge in size as a man ages. There is a risk that neoplasms may develop around the organ and result in cancerous concerns.

Pruritus Vulvae (pur-i-tus vul-vay)

Itching in the vulva.

Puerperal (pur-pur-al)

A period after childbirth to analyze the woman's functionality. The period may last for up to eight weeks after birth.

Pyometra (pie-oh-me-trah)

The development of pus in the uterine cavity.

Quickening

Fetal movements that the mother may feel. These may become prominent after the first four months of the pregnancy.

Salpingitis (sal-ping-eye-tis)

Inflammation in the fallopian tube.

Salpingostomy (sal-ping-os-toe-mee)

The development of an opening in a fallopian tube produced for surgery.

Scrotum (skroe-tum)

A pouch of skin that appears under the penile. The testicles are situated inside the scrotum.

Semen (see-min)

A thick fluid that is produced by a man following ejaculation. The semen includes the sperm and plasma that helps keep the sperm active. The compound is produced by the prostate gland.

Seminoma (see-min-oh-ma)

A malignant growth in the testis. This may require the removal of the tissue.

Sex

A general statement of the reproductive functionality of the human body. The sex is determined based on the form that the genitalia produces as well as the general hormonal production of the body.

SGA

Small for Gestational Age. This is relative to a newborn who is smaller in size than what is normal for the gestational age. This may be the bottom tenth percentile for average weight. A child who is used 3,000 grams in weight may be interpreted as being SGA.

Shaken Baby Syndrome

A condition where a child experiences brain injuries following sudden motions. The condition may be deadly. The brain injuries develop due to the child being shaken while being held by the chest or shoulders or other parts. The intense cranial motions may produce a hemorrhage, although outside signs of damage may not be visible.

Sperm

A sex cell found in the male body. This may also be referred to as a spermatozoon. The cell includes the genetic information that is to be transferred by the male to the female body for the proper fertilization of the egg.

Spermatids (spur-mah-tids)

Sperm cells that have not fully matured. These include cells that are found in the testicle.

Spermatozoa (spur-mat-oe-zoe-ah)

Male germ cells that are fully mature. These have matured from spermatids.

STD

Sexually transmitted disease. This is a condition that may be transferred from people through sexual interaction. Some STDs may be treated, while others will stay in the body for an extended period of time.

Sterile

Unable to produce a child. This may also refer to an instrument used in a procedure that is clean and safe for use.

Syphilis (sif-il-is)

A bacterial STD that develops in the body. This starts as a sore in the body and eventually spreads. The condition may be identified in stages. Stage 1 syphilis appears as a sore a few days after infection. Stage 2 syphilis is a body rash that occurs a few weeks later. Stage 3 syphilis will impact the physical organs, although that may not occur for years after the initial infestation.

TAH

Total abdominal hysterectomy. The uterus and cervix are both removed from the body through an incision in the lower abdomen.

Teratology (tear-ah-tol-o-gee)

A study of developmental issues.

Term Birth

A definition of when the childbirth process takes place after the pregnancy goes through its normal cycle. This should occur between 37 to 40 weeks after the pregnancy began.

Testicle (tess-tick-ul)

The testis and the ducts involved.

Testis (tes-tees)

A gonad situated in the scrotum. A man should have two of these.

TFS

Testicular feminization syndrome. A male fetus is not being responsive to androgens or male hormones. The testes may be found in the abdomen. A short pouch of vaginal tissue may develop, although there are no uterus, ovaries, or fallopian tubes to be found in the body.

Thecoma (thek-oe-ma)

A neoplasm that develops in the ovarian tissue.

Thelarche (thel-arch)

The development of the breast tissue during puberty.

Trichomoniasis (tick-oh-mon-ee-ah-sis)

Also called Trich A sexually transmitted disease caused by a parasitic infection. The STD is the production of vaginal discharge and itching in the female body. This may result in a risk of premature birth for a pregnant woman. Men may also develop the condition, although they may not show any distinguishable symptoms.

Trimester

A three-month period of the pregnancy.

TUR

Transurethral resection. The process treats benign prostatic hyperplasia or BPH. It is an electrocautery process conducted through the urethra to treat the condition.

Umbilicus (um-bil-i-kus)

The navel tissue. This is the area in the center of the abdominal wall where the umbilical cord connected to the fetus.

Umbilical (um-bill-ik-ul)

Referring to the opening part of the abdominal wall where blood vessels go from the placenta to other parts of the body.

Umbilical Cord

A rope-like material that connects the fetus to the placenta. The cord includes blood vessels responsible for delivering oxygen and other nutrients from the mother's body to the fetus. The tissue also eliminates waste materials from the fetus.

Uterine (you-tur-in)

Relating to the uterus.

Uterine Prolapse

An issue where the uterus drops into the vaginal area.

Uterus (you-tur-us)

The organ between the bladder and rectum. This is where the unborn child develops.

Vagina (vahj-eye-nah)

A muscular tube area that connects the uterine cervix to the vulva and the outside parts of the body.

Vaginitis (vah-gin-eye-tis)

Vaginal inflammation. A slight discharge from the vaginal region.

Varicocele (var-ik-oe-sell)

When veins in the spermatic cord become too large.

Vasectomy (vas-eck-toe-mee)

A medical procedure that causes men to become sterile. The permanent process is the vas deferens tubes being severed, thus preventing sperm from entering the semen. The sperm cells will remain in the testicles and will be absorbed by the body.

Vasovasostomy (vas-oe-vas-oe-stoe-mee)

A procedure that reverses the effects of the vasectomy. The connections in the vas deferens are restored. The man's fertility will not be fully restored, although the practice may help improve the chances of a man to produce a child.

Venereal Disease

Also called VD. A contagious condition that is transferred through sexual contact. This may be caused by a bacteria, virus, or parasite being transferred to the other sexual partner.

Vulva (vul-vah)

The external genitals on the female body. The vulva includes the labia, clitoris, and vestibule.

Vulvitis (vul-vy-tis)

Inflammation in the vulva.

WD

Well-developed. This may refer to when the body has fully developed some of its sexual functions and components.

Zygote (zie-goat)

A fertilized ovum that is produced when male and female gametes link up.

Prefixes

amni/o	ammion
andr/o	male
balan/o	glans penis
chori/o	chorion
colp/o	vagina
embryo	embryo
endometri/o	endometrium
epididym/o	epididymis
episi/o	vulva
fet/o	fetus
galact/o	milk
genit/o	reproduction
gest/o	bearing
gon	genital functions
gonad/o	sex glands
gynec/o	female
gyno	female
hymen/o	membrane
hyster/o	uterus

lact/o	milk
lacti	milk
mamm/o	breast
mast/o	breast
men/o	menstruation
metr/o	uterus
nat/o	birth
obstetr/o	obstetrics or midwifery
omphal/o	navel
oophor/o	ovary
orchid/o	testicles
osche/o	scrotum
ov/o	egg or ovum
ovari/o	ovary
perine/o	perineum
phall/o	penis
prostat/o	prostate
salping/o	fallopian tube
scrot/o	scrotum
semin/i	semen
sperm/o	sperm cells
sperma	sperm
test/I	testicle
thel/o/e	nipple
toc/o	labor and birthing

umbilic	relating to the navel
uter/o	uterus
vagin/o	vagina
varic/o	varices
venere/o	relating to sexual activities
vulv/o	vulva

Chapter 10 – Skeletal System

The skeletal system refers to the bones and other structures needed to ensure the body can stay intact. The ligaments, cartilage, and other materials in the body needed for its support are also included within the skeletal system.

Acetabulum (a-set-ahb-you-lum)

The surface on the pelvis where the head of the femur is located.

Achondroplasia (eh-chon-droe-play-ja)

A condition where a person develops short limbs. This is a form of dwarfism.

Acid Etching

The use of etching agents to prepare tooth surfaces. An agent like phosphoric acid may help roughen the surface to ensure material can adhere to the tooth properly.

Acromioclavicular Joint (eh-crome-mio-klav-ick-u-lur)

A joint on the outside part of the clavicle and the margin along the scapula. The joint includes six separate ligaments.

Acromion (eh-crow-mee-in)

The extension of the spine of the scapula. This is the highest part of the shoulder.

Amputation (am-pu-tay-shun)

The removal of a limb or other part of the body.

Ankle

An area on the lower body between the leg and foot that connects the two parts.

Ankylosis (an-kil-oh-sis)

When a joint becomes immobile.

Anodontia (ahn-oh-don-shah)

When a patient has most or all of their teeth missing. This may be a congenital condition.

Anterior Cruciate Ligament (crew-shee-it)

A knee ligament that is in the tibia and goes to the posterior area of the femur. The ACL is required for the stability of the knee, particularly during rotation.

Apophysis (eh-pop-fiss-iss)

A projection that develops out of a bone. This may also be an outgrowth that is unplanned.

Arthralgia (arth-ral-gee-ah)

Joint pain.

Arthritis (arth-rye-tis)

The inflammation of a joint. This may occur along any joint and will result in swelling. The pain involved may result in a reduced range of motion within the body part involved.

Arthrocentesis (arth-ro-sent-ee-sis)

The development of fluid in a joint cavity.

Arthrodesis (arth-ro-dee-sis)

When a joint is fixed in a surgical procedure by fusing joint surfaces together. The process is designed to promote the growth of bone cells in the targeted area.

Arthrography (arth-rog-ra-fee)

Imaging of a joint. A contrast dye is injected into the target area to improve how the area can be seen.

Arthrolysis (arth-rol-iss-iss)

A surgical routine that restores a joint that has become stiff. The goal is to enhance the mobility of the target joint.

Arthroplasty (arth-ro-plas-tee)

Surgery to rebuild a joint. The procedure helps relieve pains in the body or restore natural motion.

Arthroscopy (arth-ros-kop-ee)

An exam of a joint where an endoscope is inserted in the area to identify the condition.

Articulation

A connection between two bones. The articulation occurs in a joint.

Auranofin (or-ann-oh-fin)

A drug that helps treat rheumatoid arthritis.

Autologous (aw-toe-low-gus)

A person being both a donor and a recipient of something. This definition frequently refers to body fluids, particularly blood.

Axilla (ax-ill-ah)

The armpit region.

Bicuspid (by-kuss-pid)

A premolar tooth. The tooth is frequently used for grinding food.

Bone Mineral Density

A measure of how many minerals are found in bone tissue. The test of the BMD is typically used to identify cases of osteoporosis.

Bone Density

A measurement of bone mineral for every square centimeter of bone. The measurement may identify if a bone is developing properly or if a person is at risk of developing osteoporosis.

Brachial (brah-key-ul)

Relating to arm tissue.

Bregma (brig-mah)

A space on the top part of the cranium where the coronal and sagittal sutures meet.

Bruxism (bruks-iz-im)

A condition where a person consistently grinds their teeth; this may occur both while asleep and when awake.

Bunion (bun-e-in)

A thick tissue that appears around the metatarsal phalangeal joint. The tissue may be firm and can be caused by repeated motions. The issue occurs mainly in the big toe area.

Bursa (burr-sah)

A fluid sac located near a joint. The sac protects the moving parts around muscles, tendons, or other tissues in the body.

Bursitis (burr-sigh-tis)

Inflammation in a bursa.

Calcaneus (cal-sane-e-nus)

A large tarsal bone located on the back part of the foot. The bone is necessary for forming the heel.

Capsulitis (cap-sue-lie-tis)

Inflammation of a capsule around a joint.

Carpal (car-pull)

A condition involving the wrist.

Carpal Bone (car-pull bone)

A bone located in the wrist. These bones include the scaphoid, lunate, pisiform, trapezium, triquetrum, capitate, hamate, and trapezoid bones.

Cartilage (car-ti-lige)

Connective tissues that are responsible for keeping joints together. The tissue is non-vascular and is secured in a single matrix.

Cerclage (sur-kl-ige)

When the ends of a bone fracture are secured. This may also include securing any bone chips that might have formed around different parts of the body, most notably the patella.

Cervical Region (sur-vik-ul)

The uppermost region in the spinal column. This involves the seven vertebrae in the column that connect to the neck area. The region makes up the bones for the neck. The seven vertebrae are labeled as C1 to C7. A break in the vertebrae may result in the most significant form of paralysis in a patient.

Chondral (kon-drul)

Relating to cartilage.

Chondrocyte (kon-dro-cite)

A cell that produces cartilage.

Chondrogenesis (kon-dro-gen-eh-sis)

The production of cartilage.

Chondroma (kon-dro-ma)

A tumor that is formed from the cells that produce cartilage. The tumor is usually benign.

Chondromalacia (kon-dro-mal-a-see-ah)

The breakdown of cartilage, including the softening of the tissue. The condition frequently happens in the knees and is common among those who are physically active in that area.

Chondrosarcoma (kon-dro-sar-koh-ma)

A malignant growth of cartilage cells. The condition occurs mainly in the pelvic bones or scapula.

Clavicle (klav-ickl)

The collar bone connected to the shoulders These bones are found closer to the neck and are often visible under the skin.

Clubfoot

A condition where the foot is deformed so that the person is unable to stand with the sole flat on the ground.

Coccygeal Region (cock-eh-gee-ul)

The lowest section of the spinal column along the coccyx or tailbone. The area initially features four vertebrae listed from C1 to C4. Over time, the points will fuse together to create a single bone. The fusion takes place prior to adulthood.

Collagen (kol-ah-gin)

A protein that produces skin, cartilage, and other tissues. Collagen ensures the skin can flex and will not produce wrinkles.

Costochondritis (cost-oh-kon-dry-tis)

Inflammation in the costal cartilage. The issue develops mainly when a person uses their chest muscles too often.

Cranial (kray-nee-ul)

Involving the cranium.

Cranium (kray-nee-um)

The skeletal part of the head. The area keeps the brain in its place.

Crepitation (krep-it-tay-shun)

The cracking sound that often develops in joints.

Cubital (cue-bit-ul)

Relating to the elbow or forearm.

Cuspid (cus-pid)

A tooth that has one cusp. This is the third tooth to either side of the midline on the jaw.

Dactylitis (dak-til-eye-tis)

Inflammation in the fingers and toes.

Degenerative Joint Disease

A form of arthritis that develops when tissues along the end parts of the bones wear down. The condition is also known as osteoarthritis.

Dentin (den-tin)

The surface that forms teeth. The compound is secured by enamel and cementum on the outside of the tooth.

Dislocation

When a body part is displaced from its normal position. The condition is most frequently used to discuss a joint.

Enarthrosis (en-ar-throw-sis)

A ball and socket joint.

Endomorph (en-doe-morf)

A body that has a soft feeling to it. The body is usually round.

Epineural (ep-in-ur-al)

A location located on a vertebra.

Exoskeleton (ex-oh-skel-i-ton)

An outside structure or shell. This may be found in some parts of the body, although the term typically refers to the protective structure that is found in the form of a shell.

Exostoses (ex-oh-stoe-sis)

An unusual outgrowth from the bone's surface. The outgrowth has a bony feeling.

Femur (fee-mur)

A long bone found between the hip and knee. This is the longest bone in the human body.

Flexion (flex-e-in)

The process where a person bends a limb. This may also refer to the position that the limb takes when it is bent.

Forearm (four-arm)

A part of the arm from the elbow to the wrist.

Frontal Bone

The bone on the front part of the skull.

Genu Varum (gen-oo var-um)

A slant found in the thigh. In this case, the knees are wide apart while the ankles are close together.

Glenoid Cavity (glen-oyd)

A cavity in the scapular that connects to the head of the humerus.

Gout

A form of arthritis that is caused by the development of excess uric acid crystals in the body. The condition causes swelling in the joints. The issue happens mainly in the feet, although it can be found in other parts of the body.

Hallux Valgus (hal-ucks val-gus)

A bunion.

Hemarthrosis (he-mar-throw-sis)

Bleeding that is into the joints.

Humerus (hue-mur-us)

The bone from the elbow to shoulder in the arm.

Hypertosis (high-pur-toe-sis)

When the bone starts to grow or thicken too much.

Ilium (il-ee-um)

A large bone found in the pelvic area. This is the largest and uppermost bone in the pelvic region.

Incisor (in-size-er)

A sharp tooth with a deep edge. This may be one of the maxillary or mandibular teeth.

Ischium (ish-ee-um)

The inferior area on the hip bone.

Joint Capsule

A sac found around a joint. The tissue features an outside fiber capsule and an inside synovial membrane.

Juvenile Rheumatoid Arthritis

A form of arthritis that occurs in children. The condition causes stiffness and inflammation in the joints. The condition may be diagnosed if the issue has persisted for at least six weeks.

Kyphosis (ky-foe-sis)

A change in the spinal column where the vertebral column becomes misplaced. The condition may cause the patient to constantly hunch their back.

Lacuna (la-coo-nah)

Depression found in the body.

Lamina (lam-e-nah)

A segment on the vertebral arch. The area forms the top part of the spinal canal.

Laminectomy (lam-in-eck-toe-mee)

A process where the lamina is removed or a part is removed.

Lordosis (lore-doe-sis)

An unusual curve in the lower spine. This may also be referred to as swayback.

Lumbago (lume-bah-go)

Lower back pain. The issue may not be persistent.

Lumbar Region (lum-bar)

The lower back area over the sacral vertebrae but under the thoracic vertebrae. This is the middle region of the spinal column. This includes five vertebrae listed from L1 to L5. These are the largest vertebrae. These can also handle more weight than other tissues in the area.

Macrocephaly (mack-roe-sef-alee)

Having a large head.

Malleolus (mal-ee-oh-lus)

A bony development that appears along the sides of the ankle.

Malocclusion (mal-oh-clue-shun)

When the upper and lower teeth are unable to connect with each other when the jaw is closed.

Malunion (mal-ue-nee-un)

The improper alignment of broken bone areas.

Mandible (man-di-bul)

A large bone that supports the lower teeth. The bone forms the lower jaw.

Manubrium (man-ue-bree-um)

The top area of the sternum.

Maxilla (max-il-ah)

A bone that helps to produce the upper jaw.

Maxillofacial (max-il-oh-fay-shul)

Relating to the face.

Mediastinal (mee-de-ah-stin-ul)

Relating to the median septum or another area in between two parts of the body.

Meniscus (men-is-kus)

A form of cartilage found in the knee. The tissue has a curved shape. The body will stabilize the knee joint and absorb shocks.

Metacarpals (met-ah-car-pulls)

Long bones found in the hands between the fingers and carpal bones.

Metatarsals (met-ah-tar-suls)

Long bones found in the metatarsus. These support the tarsal bones and parts that connect to the toes.

Metatarsalgia (met-ah-tar-sal-gee-ah)

Pain in the metatarsus area.

Metatarsus (met-ah-tar-sus)

An area in the foot located between the toes and the tarsus.

Microdontia (my-crow-don-tee-ah)

Small teeth.

Micrognathism (my-crow-gna-thi-sm)

A small jaw.

Molar (mo-lur)

The posterior teeth found on the jaw. These are designed for grinding.

Nasion (nay-shun)

Part on the skull where the top part of the nose connects to the forehead.

Occipital Bone

A bone that produces the back rear area of the skull.

Odontogenesis (oh-don-to-gen-e-sis)

The development of teeth.

Oligodontia (ol-eh-go-don-tee-ah)

The absence of teeth. A few teeth may be missing. The condition may be specified by mentioning particular teeth.

Open Reduction Internal Fixation

A surgical procedure used to fix a broken bone. The process requires the area to be aligned properly while a series of plates, pins, or other materials are installed to keep the bone in its place. The process helps promote the natural formation of new bone tissue provided that the fixtures are in their proper place for a prescribed time.

Orbit

A bony area in the face that holds the eyeball and other tissues involved.

Orthodontics (or-though-don-tis)

A dental procedure that corrects issues involved with the teeth. This includes using external materials to adjust how the teeth are aligned.

Orthopedics (or-thoe-pee-dix)

A surgical procedure to correct the alignment of joints and other parts of the skeletal system. This includes aligning the tissues and positioning them to allow the body to handle movement properly.

Orthotic

A device that helps with correcting orthopedic issues. Most orthotics are designed for the foot area.

Osteitis (os-tay-eye-tis)

Inflammation in the bone.

Osteoarthritis (os-tee-oh-arth-ry-tis)

Degeneration in the joints.

Osteoblastoma (os-tee-oh-blas-toe-ma)

A tumor found in the osteoid tissue or other bone structure. The tumor is painful but benign.

Osteochondritis (os-tee-oh-chon-dry-tis)

Inflammation in a bone that expands to the cartilage.

Osteochondroma (os-tee-oh-kon-droe-ma)

A tumor in the cartilage that may appear like a stalk on a bone structure. The tumor is benign in nature.

Osteochondrosis (os-tee-oh-kon-droe-sis)

A concern where the growth factors of bones may be impacted. The condition is prominent among children, although it may also be found in some adults.

Osteocytes (os-tee-oh-sites)

Osteoblasts that adhere inside of the bone matrix.

Osteogenesis (os-tee-oh-gen-i-sis)

The development of bones in the body.

Osteolysis (os-tee-oh-lye-sis)

The destruction of bone.

Osteoma (os-tee-oh-mah)

A tumor that consists of bone tissue and is benign.

Osteomalacia (os-tee-oh-mal-a-kee-ah)

Also called rickets. When the organic bone matrix stops developing.

Osteonecrosis (os-tee-oh-neck-roe-sis)

The death of a bone or a part of that tissue.

Osteophyte (os-tee-oh-fite)

A projection around joints that is a sign of arthritis. The tissue may have a bony surface.

Osteoporosis (os-tee-oh-pour-oh-sis)

When bone mass declines while the bone structure remains in the same. The condition causes fractures to develop although the tissue may appear the same on the outside.

Osteosclerosis (os-tee-skler-oh-sis)

The hardening of bone tissue. This is noticed by the tissue developing an enhanced density.

Palate (pal-at)

A structure that is formed around the roof of the mouth. The anterior hard palate and posterior soft palate keep the structure intact.

Paratenon (par-ah-tin-on)

A tissue that develops between a tendon and the sheath.

Parietal Bone (par-ee-et-ul)

A quadrilateral bone that appears between the frontal and occipital bones. The bones form to produce the two sides of the cranium.

Patella (pah-tel-ah)

Also called the kneecap. A bone located on the front part of the knee.

Pelvis (pel-vis)

A lower part of the abdomen. It is a bone structure that is supported by the hip bones. The sacrum and coccyx also help keep the tissue in its place.

Periarthritis (pear-ee-ar-th-rye-tis)

Inflammation in the tissues around a joint.

Periosteum (pear-ee-oh-stee-um)

A membrane that covers the surface part of a bone with the exception of the articular cartridge and other areas where the bone connects to ligaments and tendons.

Periostitis (pear-ee-oh-sty-tis)

Inflammation in the periosteum.

Phalangitis (fal-ange-eye-tis)

Inflammation in a finger or toe.

Proximal Interphalangeal (in-tur-phal-an-gee-al)

Also called PIP. This is the third bone on a finger. The bone is below the intermediate phalange and ahead of the metacapsule. The PIP supports the connection of one of the top joints in a finger.

Plagiocephaly (plah-ge-oh-sef-al-ee)

When a person develops a flat area on the head. This is common in newborns and may occur when the baby lies on its back for too long. The condition will not cause brain damage nor will it negatively influence a child's development. The issue may be controlled by changing the baby's position when sleeping or lying. A molded helmet may also be required for treatment if the child's head does not improve in appearance before the age of four.

Plantar (plan-tur)

The bottom part of the foot.

Platybasia (plat-ee-bay-shah)

A misshapen cranium. The skull base is flat. The posterior cranial fossa is upward around the foramen magnum.

Polyarthritis

When a person experiences inflammation or arthritis in many joints.

Polychondritis (pol-e-con-dry-tis)

Inflammation of cartilage.

Polydactyly (pol-e-dack-tyl-ee)

When a person's hand or foot has more fingers or toes than normal. The excess fingers or toes are called supernumerary digits. The condition is genetic and may be transmitted between family members. The need to remove these added fingers or toes will vary based on how they have formed and if these tissues are impacting a person's functionality.

Popliteal (pop-lit-eel)

Relating to the area behind the knee.

Precordium (pree-kord-ee-um)

A part of the thorax over the heart tissue.

Pseudarthrosis (sue-dar-throw-sis)

A fibrous joint that develops on an unhealed fracture. The area is not an actual joint, but it may have the motion of a joint. This is an area of the bone structure that has not fully healed following an injury or surgical procedure.

Psoriatic Arthritis (sore-ee-at-ik)

Arthritis that is paired with psoriasis. The condition impacts joints and the spinal column.

Pubic Bone (pue-bick)

A bone that is found in the lower part of the hip bones. The bone surrounds the pubic region of the body.

Pubic Symphysis

A joint that develops between the pubic bones. The joint appears below the urinary bladder.

Pyarthrosis (pie-ar-throw-sis)

Inflammation of the synovial membrane. The condition develops when a joint experiences a bacterial infection. The issue may be diagnosed by taking a sample of fluid from the joint and examining the tissue.

Range of Motion

An analysis of how well a person is capable of moving their joints and other body parts. The ROM may be analyzed to determine if a person has arthritis or another condition. This may also identify the intensity of an injury, although proper safeguards may be required to prevent the impact from becoming worse.

Rheumatoid Factor (rue-mah-toid)

Also called RF. The factor may be found in cases where a person has rheumatoid arthritis and other autoimmune diseases. A blood test may identify the RF count. The ideal count for the body should be under 15 IU per milliliter of blood sampled.

Rheumatic (rue-mat-ick)

A disorder that influences joints and other connective tissues. The most common rheumatic issues include degenerative and inflammatory concerns.

Rheumatoid Arthritis

Also called RA. The autoimmune condition will trigger pain and swelling in the joints. The tissues may feel stiff. The joints will not experience a full range of motion. The hands and wrists are the areas most likely to develop RA.

Ribs

Curved bones that cover the chest organs. The ribs protect the chest. The ribs include twelve curved bones that connect to the vertebral column and will form costal cartilage. Some people may have an added curved bone, although this may not be a sign of anything significant.

Rickets (rick-its)

Also called osteomalacia. A disease where the bones are unable to mineralize. Rickets is triggered by a lack of vitamin D, calcium, or phosphate. The disease will cause the bones to become unable to develop properly. A patient may develop bow legs and pains in the bones as well as general weakness in the bone tissues.

Sacral Region (sac-rul)

The spinal column region located under the lumbar vertebrae. This is the fourth of the spinal column regions and is the second-to-lowest one. The column includes five vertebrae from S1 to S5. The child's body will mature and eventually allow the bones to fuse together to develop as the sacrum.

Sacroiliitis (sack-roe-il-ee-eye-tis)

Inflammation in the sacroiliac joint. The disorder triggers lower back pain and a fever as well as a decreased range of motion.

Sacrum (sack-rum)

A triangular bone found on the dorsal section of the pelvis. The bone appears between the hip bones. The sacrum supports the pelvis and keeps it stable.

Sagittal (saj-it-ul)

A plane that goes down the long axis in the body. The plane is parallel to the median plane. The sagittal plane may be used to identify how well the body moves and how it can flex.

Scaphoid Bone (scaf-oid)

A small bone found in the wrist. The bone is the most lateral in the carpal bones.

Scapula (scap-ue-lah)

The shoulder blade. The bone is found in the back part of the shoulder. This is flat and triangular in appearance.

Scoliosis (skoe-lee-oh-sis)

A sideway curve that appears in the spine. The curve appears prior to puberty. The curve may cause intense pains, although it is not likely to produce paralysis. A brace may be required to control the curve, and surgery may be necessary in the most intense cases.

Sesamoid (sez-ah-moid)

A small bone that develops in a tendon. The bone will develop when it moves over an angular structure in the body. The kneecap is an example.

Shoulder

A connection where the clavicle, scapula, and humerus link together. The shoulder is where the arm connects to the remaining part of the body.

Shoulder Dislocation

When the humerus is removed from the scapula. This may not be a fracture or break, although this may cause intense pains and a loss of sensation.

Skeleton

The series of bones that will form the body. The skeleton is responsible for protecting the body and ensuring all organs and tissues are secured.

Skull

The skeletal part of the head. The skull includes the bones that will protect the brain and form the person's facial features.

Sling

A bandage used to support an injured part of the body. The sling immobilizes the body part to ensure the tissue will not be impacted when it is healing.

Sphenoid Bone (sfen-oid)

An irregular bone found at the base of the skull. The bone appears between the frontal, temporal, and occipital bones.

Spina Bifida (spy-na bif-eh-da)

A birth defect also called a split spine. The membranes around the spinal cord do not close completely. The condition develops mainly in the lower back, although in rare cases it can appear at a higher part of the spinal column. The vertebrae does not function properly and cause spinal fluid to develop in the cord and nerves. Spinal tissue may start to protrude due to the issue. Surgery is needed to close the membranes. Muscle weakness may develop due to this condition.

Spine

A large column of vertebrae down the center of a person's back. The spinal column is needed to convey motions in the body and to support the central nervous system. Any breaks in the spinal column may result in paralysis.

Spondylitis (spon-dyl-eye-tis)

Inflammation in the synovial joints in the back.

Spondylolisthesis (spon-dyl-oh-lis-tee-sis)

When the vertebra in the base of the spine slips. The bone will slip forward onto the bone below the impacted one. The injury may develop when a person engages in repetitive actions that put stress on the bones in the area. Genetics may also be a factor. The vertebra may slip far enough to cause intense back pains as the tissue presses on a nerve. This may also cause nerve crowding, a problem that causes extreme pains or numbness in the leg. Rest is required in most cases, although surgery is required if the problem does correct itself after some time.

Spondylosis (spon-dil-oh-sis)

A degenerative condition that will become worse as a person gets older. This is a form of osteoarthritis that develops in the spine. The condition can develop in any part of the spine. A disc may become thin and eventually trigger bone spurs. Those who are older will have a higher risk of spondylosis. Medications may be used, but the condition does not have any full cures.

Sternoclavicular Joint (stur-noe-clav-ick-u-lur)

A double gliding joint that forms in the clavicle. This is the area where the clavicle connects to the manubrium in the sternum.

Sternum (stur-num)

A flat bone called the breastbone. The bone appears in the midsection of the anterior thoracic region or chest region. The sternum stabilizes the rib cage and supports many other muscles responsible for supporting the arms, head, and neck.

Subtalar Joint (sub-tal-ar)

A joint produced by the connection of the talus and calcaneus.

Synovectomy (sign-oh-vec-toe-mee)

The removal of the membrane or synovium that lines a joint. The surgical procedure is for cases where the body experiences regular inflammation. The knee is the most prominent part of the body that a synovectomy may be performed.

Talus (tal-us)

A large ankle bone. The bone connects to the tibia and the calcaneum and navicular bones.

Tarsal (tar-sul)

Relating to the bones in the ankle and foot.

Tarsal Bones

The bones that produce the tarsus.

Tarsal Joints

Connections between each of the tarsal bones.

Tarsalgia (tar-sal-ja)

Pain in the foot. The pain may be produced by irritation in the muscles or joints.

Tarsus (tar-sis)

Bones in the ankle and the proximal region of the foot.

Taxis

When a body moves back to its original position after the tissue was influenced by a fracture, dislocation, or hernia.

Temporal Bone (tem-por-ul)

One of the compound bones found in the lateral surfaces and base parts of the skull. The bones support the hearing organs.

Temporomandibular Joint (tem-por-oh-man-dib-ue-lur)

Also known as TMJ. This is one of two joints that connect the jawbone to the skull. TMJ may also refer to a condition where the joint experiences intense pains and impaired jaw movements due to the surrounding muscles not working properly.

Tendinitis (ten-din-eye-tis)

Inflammation in a tendon. The pain develops outside the joint and may develop in any common tendon. Tendinitis is more likely to develop in the shoulders, knees, elbows, wrists, or heels. Athletes and others who frequently use certain body parts are most likely to be affected. Among the more common types of tendinitis include tennis elbow (forearm muscle connecting to the elbow), golfer's elbow (inner side of the elbow), swimmer's shoulder (around the shoulder blade) and Achilles tendinitis (Achilles tendon).

Tendinosis (ten-din-oh-sis)

The degeneration of collagen in a tendon. The condition occurs due to a person using the same tendon many times over. The injury develops due to intense strains and requires the patient to rest.

Tendon (ten-din)

A series of white fibrous tissues. The connective tissue connects the muscle to a bone.

Tenodesis (ten-oh-dee-sis)

A process where biceps tendonitis in the shoulder is treated. The biceps tendon will be secured through passive tension to ensure the development of the tissue.

Tenoplasty (ten-oh-plas-tee)

The surgical repair of a tendon.

Tenosynovitis (ten-oh-sin-ohv-eye-tis)

Inflammation in the synovium, a fluid sheath that surrounds the tendon. The inflammation causes joint pains and swelling along with some stiffness. The condition may be treated through pain relievers and by immobilizing the impacted joint. Corticosteroid injections may be required in some of the more intense situations.

Tenotomy (ten-aw-toe-mee)

When a tendon is surgically opened. The opening is used to reshape the tendon. The procedure is used mainly for treating club foot-related concerns. The Achilles tendon is often the most likely area to be impacted by the procedure.

Thoracic Region (thor-as-ick)

The second-highest region on the spinal column. This is the spinal tissues in the chest area. The twelve vertebrae in the thoracic region can be listed as T1 to T12 or as D1 to D12. Each of the vertebrae is connected to a rib.

THR

Total hip replacement. The procedure replaces a hip joint that is damaged or fully worn. The old joint is replaced with a prosthetic joint. The bone and cartilage that has worn are removed and replaced. The femoral head is removed and replaced with a new compound added in the center part of the femur. Metal materials may be used in the prosthesis. The THR process is used for cases when a person has intense arthritis in the hip that is not being treated by other procedures. The procedure is also used when a person has experienced a hip fracture and the tissue cannot heal on its own.

Tibia (tib-ee-ah)

The large body in the lower leg. The bone connects laterally to the fibula.

TKR

Total knee replacement. The surgical procedure is for cases where the knee is experiencing intense arthritis and other treatments have failed. This includes cases of osteoarthritis, rheumatoid arthritis, and psoriatic arthritis. The replacement may also help in cases where a person has experienced a significant fracture or another form of damage to the knee joint. Metal materials with some plastics replace the thighbone and shinbone. A high-density plastic compound is applied as a substitute to the cartilage along with the artificial bone compounds.

Ulna (ul-nah)

An inner bone in the forearm. This is the longer of the two bones in the forearm.

Ulnar (ul-nar)

Relating to the ulna.

Vertebrae (vur-teh-bray)

A small bone that is part of the backbone. Each vertebra includes projections to support the muscles. A hole is found in each bone to allow the spinal cord to pass through. The vertebrae include (from top to bottom) seven cervical, twelve thoracic, five lumbar, five sacrum, and four coccyx vertebrae. Damages to any of these vertebrae may cause paralysis in the body with the paralysis being based on the type of damage that develops.

Xiphoid (zip-oid)

An extension in the lower or inferior segment of the sternum.

Zygoma (zy-goe-mah)

A pair of bones that support the cheek and the orbit on either side of the skull.

Important Prefixes and Roots

ankyl	bent
arthr	joint
articul/o	joint
axi/o	axis
brachi	arm
burs/o	bursa

calc	calcium
calcane	heel
carp/o	wrist
caud	tail
centr	center
cephal	head
cervic	neck or cervix
cheir	hand
chir	hand
chondr/i/o	cartilage
clavicul	clavicle
cleid	clavicle
coccyg	coccyx
condy	knob
cost/o	rib
crani	skull
cubit	elbow or forearm
dactyl/o	fingers and toes
digit/o	finger or toe
drom/o	running
faci	face
femor	femur
geni	chin
genu	knee
gnath	cheek or jaw

goni	angle
ili/o	ilium
ithy	erect or straight
kyph	bent
lamin	lamina
lord	curve
lox	slant
lumb	lower back
mandibul	mandible
mastoid	bone behind the ear
maxilla	upper jawbone
mel/o	limb
noto	back
om	shoulder
opsith	behind
oss/e/i	bone
oste/o	bone
petr/o	hard
pod/o	foot
rachi/o	spinal column
sacr/o	sacrum
scapul/o	scapula
scoli/o	curved
sphenoid/o	sphenoid
spin/o	spine

spondyl/o	vertebra
stern/o	sternum
synovi/o	synovial joint
tal/o	ankle
tars/o	ankle or tarsal bone
tib/I	tibia
xiph/o	xiphoid

Chapter 11 – Urinary System

The urinary system refers to the urinary tract and its general functionality. The system is studied in the field of urology with a focus on the analysis and treatment of conditions relating to the urinary tract in both men and women. This includes an analysis of the genital tract in the male body.

The urinary system is also referred to as the renal system.

The urinary system includes the kidneys, bladder, urethra, and ureters. The system removes excess waste from the body while also controlling electrolyte and metabolite levels in the body. Blood pH levels are also controlled through the support of the urinary or renal system.

Ablation (ab-lay-shin)

The removal of tissue in the urinary area. This may be done through freezing or vaporization among other methods.

Anuria (an-ur-ee-ah)

When urine does not form.

ART

Acute renal failure. This is a condition of the renal system failing to function.

Bladder

A muscular sac that secures urine that is produced by the kidneys. The sac will continue to hold the urine until the person excretes it via the urinary tract.

Blood Urea Nitrogen

A review of the amount of urea in the blood.

Calyx (cal-icks)

A chamber in the kidney that urine passes through. The plural form is calyces. Many of these calyces will connect together to help move urine through the renal pelvis and eventually to the uterer.

Cystitis (sist-eye-tis)

Inflammation in the urinary bladder.

Cystocele (sis-to-cell)

A prolapse of the bladder in the female body. The bladder will move into the vaginal area.

Dialysis (dye-al-i-sis)

A procedure used in patients who have experienced kidney or renal failure. A process is a form of therapy responsible for removing harmful wastes and fluids in the blood.

Diuresis (dy-ur-ee-sis)

An increase in the production and removal of urine.

Endometrium (en-doh-mee-tree-um)

A coating of the inside layer of the uterine wall. The tissue should thicken and restore on its own to prepare for a pregnancy. The area may also take in the embryo for conception. The endometrium will shed some of its tissues over time during menstrual processes, although this will not happen if the woman is pregnant.

Enuresis (en-u-ree-sis)

The unintended discharge of urine. The discharge is involuntary and may be indicative of an underlying issue in the body.

Epispadias (ep-is-pad-ee-as)

Improper development of the urethra. The condition is a birth defect.

ERFB

Effective renal blood flow.

ESRD

End-stage rental disease. The patient's kidneys will have failed so that the person can no longer survive unless they undergo regular dialysis or have a kidney transplant.

Glomerular Filtration Rate (glom-er-ue-lur)

A test used to identify how well the kidneys function. The test analyzes the amount of blood that passes through the glomeruli in one minute.

Glomerulus (glow-mear-ue-lus)

A series of blood capillaries in the kidney. The capillaries are responsible for allowing the nephron within the kidney to stay functional. The plural form is glomeruli.

Glycosuria (gl-eye-koh-sur-ee-ah)

The development of a large amount of glucose in the urine.

Hematuria (hee-mah-tur-ee-ah)

The development of red blood cells in the urine.

Hemodialysis (hee-moh-dye-al-iss-iss)

A process that involves the removal of harmful fluids within the blood. The process is used for those who have experienced kidney failure.

Hydronephrosis (high-dro-nef-roe-sis)

The kidney becoming enlarged. The condition develops when the uterer experiences a blockage.

Hypercalciuria (high-per-kal-see-ur-ee-ah)

The presence of an elevated level of calcium in the urine.

Hyperkalemia (high-per-kal-eem-ee-ah)

A high level of potassium in the blood. The condition may develop due to acute renal failure.

Hyperoxaluria (high-per-oh-acks-ur-ee-ah)

The development of high amounts of oxalate in the urine.

Hypospadias (high-poe-spad-ee-as)

A birth defect in the urethra. The opening appears below its normal location.

Ileal

A concern relating to the ileum, a part of the small intestine that connects the jejunum and cecum.

Incontinence

A patient's inability to control how urine flows from the bladder. The issue may include either a person being unable to urinate at the right time or a person urinating when one does not intend to do so.

Intermittency

An issue in the urinary tract where the urine flow does not stay constant. The flow may start and stop at varying points during an episode resulting in incomplete emptying of the bladder.

Interstitial Cystitis (sis-tie-tis)

A condition where the bladder experiences intense pains on occasion.

Intravenous Pyelogram (pie-loh-gram)

An x-ray that examines the urinary system. The process requires iodinated contrast material to be injected intravenously. The x-ray will identify the region as the contrast compound makes the area easier to see on the review.

Ketonuria (kay-tun-ur-ee-ah)

The development of ketones in the urine.

Kidney

An organ that filters blood to allow for urine to be removed from the body. The kidney also helps regulate ion totals in the body. A person is expected to normally have two kidneys in the body.

Lithotomy (lith-ah-toe-mee)

The surgical removal of a stone or calculus from the urinary tract, kidney, or bladder.

Lymphuria (lim-fur-ee-ah)

Lymph compounds found in a person's urine.

Methenamine (meth-en-ah-mean)

An antibacterial drug used to treat urinary tract infections.

Nephritis (neph-rye-tis)

Inflammation in a part of the kidney.

Nephrolithiasis (neph-ro-lih-thigh-a-sis)

The development of kidney stones. A stone is also called calculus.

Nephron (nef-ron)

A small series of filtering compounds in the kidneys that are required for eliminating toxins in the blood.

Nephrosclerosis (nef-roe-skler-oh-sis)

Hardening of the kidney due to fibrous tissue developing in the area. The condition often occurs due to hypertension that is left untreated. The issue may cause the kidneys to function improperly.

Nephrosis (nef-roe-sis)

A disease that causes destruction to the kidney.

Nephrotic Syndrome (nef-rot-ick)

A condition where the kidney develops a disease in spite of no inflammatory or cancerous issues developing.

Nocturia (nock-tur-ee-ah)

When the patient has to wake up at night to urinate.

Nocturnal Enuresis (n-ur-ee-sis)

When a person involuntary urinates while sleeping at night. The condition may develop even if that person has the ability to control their urinary system.

Nonprotein Nitrogen

The urea, ammonia, and other compounds that may be found in the urinary system. These compounds are not proteins, but they can be converted into proteins by microbes within the stomach.

Oliguria (ole-eh-gur-ee-ah)

A decline in the body's ability to produce urine.

Perinephritis (pear-een-ef-rye-tis)

Inflammation in the tissues that surround the kidney. These include adipose and connective tissues.

Peritoneal Dialysis (pear-it-on-ee-al)

Dialysis that occurs when a fluid is added into the peritoneal cavity and then removed.

Phenylketonuria (fen-ill-kee-ton-ur-ee-ah)

A birth defect where phenylalanine builds up. The amino acid may develop in the body causing possible intellectual or behavioral concerns. PKU may be treated with a diet that has a limited amount of protein.

Polycystic Kidney Disease (pol-ee-sis-tick)

When cysts build up in the kidneys. The condition is inherited.

Polyuria (pol-ee-ur-ee-ah)

When the body produces an excess amount of urine.

Prostatism (pro-state-izm)

When the body slowly removes urine. The measurement may be slower when compared to how people might normally eliminate urine.

Prostatitis (pra-stat-eye-tis)

Inflammation in the male prostate gland.

Pyelectasis (pie-lec-tay-sis)

Dilation of the pelvis of the kidney.

Pyelitis (pile-eye-tis)

Inflammation in the renal pelvis.

Pyleocystitis (pile-ee-o-sist-eye-tis)

Inflammation in the kidney pelvis. The inflammation may spread to the bladder.

Pyelonephritis (pie-loh-nef-rye-tis)

Inflammation in the kidney that includes the nephrons, kidney, pelvis, and other surrounding conditions.

Pyonephrosis (pie-o-nef-roe-sis)

The kidney becoming distended due to pus and other fluids building in the area. This may cause some of the kidney tissues to become destroyed. Parts of the renal system may also become obstructed due to the condition.

Pyuria (pie-ur-ee-ah)

White blood cells forming in the urine. Some bits of pus may also appear.

Renal (ren-ul)

A condition that refers to the kidneys and how they function.

Renal Pelvis

A segment in the kidney where a series of calyces connect to one another. The pelvis is found in the middle part of the organ.

Urea (yur-ee-ah)

A compound that is produced in the liver. The compound is a nitrogen-based material that is produced after proteins are consumed. The material is usually removed from the body, although it may develop and build up in uremia.

Uremia (yur-em-ee-ah)

The development of excess urea in the blood. The issue suggests that the kidneys have failed to function properly.

Ureter (yur-et-er)

A pair of tubes that move urine from the kidney pelvis to the bladder.

Ureteral (yur-ee-tur-al)

A condition that relates to the ureter.

Ureterocele (yur-ee-tur-roe-sell)

A cyst that develops at the end of a ureter. The growth appears when the ureter moves towards the urinary bladder. The obstruction will prevent urine from flowing as necessary.

Ureterolithiasis (yur-ter-oh-lith-eye-a-sis)

The development of stones or cysts in the ureter.

Ureterostomy (yur-eter-os-toe-mee)

When a surgeon creates an opening in the ureter. The procedure is to help drain the body of urine.

Urethra (yur-ee-thra)

A tube that tranfers urine from the bladder to outside of the body. The urethra appears through the penile tissue in men and the vaginal tissue in women. The urethra is also used by the male as a portal where sperm may travel from the penile area.

Urethritis (yur-eeth-rye-tis)

Inflammation in the urethra. The condition causes pains upon urination. The flow of urine may also be difficult to manage.

Urinalysis (ur-in-al-eh-sis)

A test of the urine. The urinalysis is a review of how certain compounds respond to urine. The test identifies possible infections or other kidney disorders. The appearance of the urine may be examined alongside the concentration of the urine and how long it takes for the patient to produce the urine in the test.

Urinary Bladder

A membrane sac that appears along the urinary tract. The sac will store urine until the person engages in urination.

Urinary Catheter

A catheter that is placed into the urinary bladder or kidney. The catheter assists in removing the excess urine and other toxins from the body.

Urinary Fistula (fis-tue-lah)

An unusual passage of a part of the urinary tract. The passage may be a change between itself and with other organs.

Urinary Tract Infection

An infection that can develop in the bladder, kidney, or another part of the urinary system. The condition causes pains in the pelvic area. Women are more likely to develop the issue.

Urination

The process where a person removes urine from the body through the urethra. The urine exits the bladder after having been filtered by the kidneys.

Urine (yur-in)

The fluid that is produced by the kidneys and then secured in the bladder until urination. The fluid contains waste materials and water.

Urochesia (yur-oh-chess-ee-ah)

When urine moves through the rectum instead of through the urethra.

Urolith (yur-oh-lith)

A stone found in the urinary tract.

Urolithiasis (yur-oh-lye-thee-a-sis)

The development of stones around the urinary tract. The stones are likely to occur in the kidney or urinary bladder, although they may also appear in the ureter.

Urothelium (yur-oh-thee-lee-um)

The lining in the urinary tract

Uterer (you-tur-rur)

A series of muscle fibers around the kidneys that help to move urine from the kidneys to the bladder. These fibers allow the bladder to accept the urine that has to be removed by the body.

Prefixes

calcul	stone
cali	calyx
cupr	copper
cyst/o	urinary bladder or cyst
glomerul/o	glomerulus
lith/o	stone
nephr	kidney
pyel/o	renal pelvis
ren	kidney
ur	urine
urin	urinary system

ureter	ureter
urethr/o	urethra
vesic	bladder
vesicul	vesicle

Chapter 12 – Why Learn Medical Terms?

The medical environment that you work in will be complicated and will include many details and surroundings that will directly influence what might happen to the patients you are treating. The complexities involved are challenging, but you will have to be precise in what you are doing and expected to do as part of your job.

The medical terms you will encounter in your work will be critical to your success in treating patients. These medical terms are necessary to know for the following reasons:

- Understanding the medical condition that the patient has

- Recognizing the areas in the body that are affected by the patient's condition

- Identifying the physicalities that are associated with a condition or a part of the body

- Understanding the testing procedures that have to be used to diagnose a problem

- Knowing the procedures, surgical or otherwise, needed for treating a patient's condition

- Reviewing was has happened to a patient in the past, what may happen in the future, and what is happening to the patient at present

- Simplifying diagnoses or procedures; this includes knowing the abbreviations, acronyms, or eponyms

Such medical terms are important to ensure that everyone on a medical team understands each other and what is required for patient treatment. People who do not know the appropriate medical terms and procedures may put the patients and the medical center at risk. A lack of knowledge will cause confusion about how patients are to be treated. As a result, the wrong diagnoses or treatments may be provided to a patient, not to mention cases where diagnosis does not occur at all.

The following discusses the many reasons it is critical to understand medical terms:

1. Knowing these terms helps avoid medical errors

The most important reason why you need to learn medical terms is to ensure that you can avoid medical errors. Medical terms can be found in a patient's medical history. These terms include everything surrounding the patient's treatment needs. For instance, you might identify concerns that a patient having a history of an allergy to a certain medication. Maybe you might find information where on the patient's body the condition is impacting that person's health. You can use the appropriate medical terms to identify the problems that a patient might have.

2. Documentation is simplified.

You can also use the proper medical terms to keep the documentation accurate. In some cases, these terms may be written in full. In other cases, you might use abbreviations or acronyms for certain conditions. The simplification also ensures that the treatment ordered by the doctor can be reported in less time, thus reducing the risk for problems to develop because acronyms and abbreviations are easier to read.

3. Enhance accuracy in administering treatment.

When reading patient history reports, you can get accurate information about why a patient needs medical help and what types of treatment the patient needs or has received. The prefixes and suffixes of a word indicate the definitions.

4. Terminology is common to everyone in the workplace.

Everyone in a medical facility has to work together to ensure there is no misunderstanding associated with taking care of patients. The terminology used is common to all personnel and is universal throughout the medical community is understood by everyone dealing with medical issues.

You can use the terms in this guide to recognize the different concepts and how these terms are formed.

Chapter 13 – The Most Common Medical Terms

This guide includes an extensive array of terms that cover all the things that you might take care of when working with patients.

1. Physical Body Parts

You may have to deal with body parts and the specific regions within the body parts. For instance, you be dealing with a condition in the leg, but that condition may be on a very specific part of the leg. This could include a condition that impacts the kneecap, tibia, heel, or another area on the leg.

2. Fibers and Internal Parts

Other terms focus on certain muscle fibers, nerves, organs, and other segments inside the body. Every tissue includes several distinct parts that will influence the body.

3. Parts of Organs

Some conditions may influence certain parts of an organ. For instance, a kidney includes many parts that will directly impact how the organ functions. These include features like the ureter, cortex, and renal vein and artery. In some cases, one part of an organ will be impacted. In other instances, every part of the organ will be altered by a physical condition. Tests may identify the concerns that might develop.

4. Conditions in the Body

Individual conditions may be noticed based on the prefixes, suffixes, and root words involved. A root word may involve the part of the body that might be influenced. A root word might specify something like the type of injury or illness that is impacting the particular part of the body.

5. Diagnostic Procedures

Diagnostic procedures can be listed based on their suffixes. You may notice suffixes that focus on things like an injection or laparoscopy. You will have to know the processes of testing.

6. Treatment

Treatment includes medications and other compounds. In some cases, the treatment materials will be named for the chemical formulas of these products. In other cases, these relate to the parts of the body that they are intended to treat.

Chapter 14 – The Three Parts of a Medical Term

The parts are the prefix, the root, and the suffix. These three parts will be discussed in dedicated chapters.

1. Prefix

The prefix appears at the beginning of a word. For instance, the word "capable" means "able to do something." Adding the prefix "in" changes the meaning to the opposite of the original word.

Not all medical terms include prefixes. The prefix only identifies the number, position, or other physical quality associated with something.

2. Root

The root word is the source of the word and can be based on the Greek or Latin word for something. For instance, the word "skull" may be represented by the root word "crani" Which comes from the Greek term for "skull," which is "kranion." Understanding the Greek and Latin roots for certain physical parts of the body may help you memorize some of the root words you might encounter.

3. Suffix

The suffix is the ending of a word. Like the prefix, the letters of the suffix can directly influence the meaning of the root word. For instance, the word "ration" is "a thought or idea that may be based in sound thought." By adding the suffix "al," it becomes the word "rational," which means "sensible or logical in consideration."

A suffix can refer to various physical problems that someone might have. For instance, the suffix "algia" suggests that a person is feeling pain. The suffix "itis" means that a person is suffering from inflammation in one part of the body.

Combining the Three Parts Together

The three parts of a word can combine to produce a single term. You can use the three parts to identify how a certain medical term is introduced based on a medical condition or a type of treatment that is needed.

An example of this is the word "ultrasound" that combines two parts (the root and prefix).

1. Ultra – Outside

2. Sound – Reviewing signals based on sound waves

These two words combine to create the word "ultrasound," which refers to the use of sound waves that are applied to the outside of the body. The process is to identify certain activities that are taking place within the body.

Another example is the word "leukocytosis." This is a word that includes three parts:

1. Leuko – White

2. Cyt – Root, which is for blood cell

3. Osis – An unusual condition

Leukocytosis refers to an unusual condition where white blood cells are not forming properly. The color of the cells is introduced at the start, followed by the root of the word referring to blood cells. The suffix refers to an abnormal condition that needs to be treated based.

Chapter 15 – Pronouncing Words

One of the greatest concerns when learning medical terms is knowing the correct pronunciation.

Medical terms are notorious for having difficult pronunciations. These words include many complicated pairings of letters that can make it a challenge.

The following is a list of some of the most common considerations to use when pronouncing certain words.

Note: Many of the terms that you will encounter in this guide have the pronunciations included.

Letters	Pronunciation
j	j
sk	sk
ph	f
sc	sk
n (when a vowel follows)	n
psy	sigh
x	z
cho	k
gy	guy
gi	j
ge	j
ce	si
ci	si
kn	n
ca	k
cu	k
ph	f

cy (followed by s)	see
cy (followed by others)	si
sch	sk
n (followed by a vowel)	n
k (followed by a vowel)	k
z	z
oe	e
thy (at the beginning)	thi
ty (at the beginning)	ti
thy (at the end)	thee
ty (at the end)	tee
g (prefix)	guh
my (at the end)	me
my (at the beginning)	my
g (root followed by e or i)	j
pn	n

For instance, the word "typhoid" would be pronounced as "tie-foid" and "colorectomy" would be pronounced as "ko-lo-rec-to-mee."

The chapters in this guide include individual terms for certain body segments and how to pronounce those words correctly. Remember that the correct pronunciation is vital to ensure correct verbal communication between doctors, nurses, and others responsible for certain processes in the medical environment.

Chapter 16 – Prefixes

The general consideration surrounding prefixes is that they are used to introduce concepts about where something may be located or about other treatments that may be ordered. This chapter focuses on various prefixes that will introduce a root word.

Note: The individual chapters in this guide relating to different physical systems will include segments that feature prefixes dedicated to their fields. Refer to the end parts of those chapters to find information on those systems and how they may work.

Positional Prefixes

Positional prefixes describe a location or place in the body. Such prefixes can be used to identify where treatment is to be administered.

Prefix	Meaning
circum	around
dexi	right
endo	within or inside
epi	over or outer
hypo	below or under
infra	under
inter	between
levo	left
medi	middle
mes	middle
peri	around
post	after or behind
pre	before
pro	before
retro	behind or backward
sinister	left

sub	under or beneath
trans	across

For instance, "epidermal" refers to the outer layer of the skin. "Epi" means outside, "derm" refers to the skin, and "al" is the suffix that indicates pertaining to something..

Numerical

Numerical prefixes refer to the number of something that might be identified. This also includes how something is to be provided or the quantity that is needed. These prefixes are critical for situations like when very specific treatment procedures are required for ensuring the body is treated as necessary.

Prefix	Meaning
bi	two
dipl/o	double
hemi	half
mono	one
uni	one
multi	multiple or more than one
poly	many
prima	first
quadri	four
tri	three

An example is "quadriplegia." The condition refers to paralysis in all four limbs. "Quadri" is the prefix "plegia" is a suffix for paralysis. The word "polydactyly" refers to a person having more fingers on the hand than normal. The "poly" prefix means many and "dactyl" relates to a finger and "y" relates to a certain condition that might appear within the body.

Measurement

Measurement prefixes refer to the intensity or degree of a condition. This includes understanding how large or small something might be or whether some kind of activity will take place based on how intense or minimal the situation may be.

Prefix	Meaning
hyper	greater than normal
hypo	less than normal
macro	large
megalo	very large
micro	small

A person may experience "hypoglycemia," for instance. This means that a person has a lower than normal blood sugar level. The "hypo" prefix means less than, "gylc" for sugar and the suffix "emia" refers to a condition relating to blood.

Speed

Speed frequently refers to a procedure that takes place in the body. It could also refer to the treatment and how that treatment may work to alleviate a certain condition.

Prefix	Meaning
brady	slow
hyper	rapid
hypo	lacking
tachy	fast

"Tachycardia" refers to a condition where a person's heart rate is faster than the normal. The "tachy" prefix means fast, "cardi" is the root word relating to the heart and the suffix "a" refers to a condition.

Directional Prefixes

A directional prefix refers to the path or route that concern or treatment will follow. Some of these directional prefixes are shared with the positional prefixes. However, the directional prefixes focus on the directions that a person must take when handling a certain procedure or the directions that parts of the body may move towards or influence.

Prefix	Meaning
ab	away from
ad	toward

circum	around
dextro	right
dia	through
ecto	outside
endo	within or inside
eso	inward
exo	outward
extra	outside
intra	within
levo	left
para	near or beside
peri	around
supper	upper
trans	through
tropia	turning
ultra	beyond

For example, the word "ultrasonography" refers to an analysis of tissues that can be identified beyond what a person is capable of identifying. The prefix "ultra" refers to going beyond. The word "transvaginal" has the prefix "trans" meaning going through, so the word means going through the vaginal tissues in the body.

General Prefixes

The following prefixes focus on some of the basic concepts.

Prefix	Meaning
a	without
an	without
anti	against

auto	self
con	alongside
contra	against
de	to rid the body of
dis	to undo a natural condition
dys	improper functionality or pain
eu	well or pleasant
hemi	half
hetero	different
homo	same
homeo	similar to
idio	singular
mal	negative
pan	complete or comprehensive
pseudo	false
pathy	relating to a disease
semi	half
syn	similarity or likeness

Testing

Testing prefixes indicate the diagnostic process that will be used and the various tools that may be used on different parts of the body or tools responsible for performing the tests.

Prefix	Meaning
echo	using ultrasonic waves
electro	using electricity
endo	internal, as in an instrument going inside a part of the body

sono	the production of sound
ultra	from outside of the body; this also relates to the use of ultrasonic waves

Color

Color prefixes refer to the physical appearance. For instance, an erythrocyte refers to a red blood cell and a leukocyte refers to a white blood cell.

Note: The Greek prefixes for these words are listed first, followed by the Latin prefixes. The Greek terms are used the most often in medical terms, although Latin roots may also be used.

Root Word	Greek Root	Latin Root
black	melan	nigr
blue	cyan	cerule
gold	chrys	aur
gray	poli	can
green	chloro	vir
purple	porphyr	purpur
red	erythr	rub
reddish-orange	cirrh	
white	leuk	alb
yellow	xanth	flav (French root: jaun)

For example, "chlorophyll." The term refers to a pigment in plant materials that provides plants with nutrients while adding a green pigment. The "chloro" prefix states that the compound is green. The word "cirrhosis" refers to when the liver becomes damaged. The condition uses the "cirrh" prefix to refer to how the condition triggers the liver into becoming discolored.

Chapter 17 – Root Words

The root words typically refer to certain body parts. Root words come from Latin or Greek words.

These root words can be used to identify certain conditions that a person might have. Also, these root words could double as prefixes to indicate a body part.

Not all words have both Greek and Latin roots. Some of these words also have some roots from different languages. For instance, the roots "nephron" and "ren" both relate to the kidney. These can combine to produce words with "nephritis" or "renal failure" among other terms relating to how the kidney functions.

Describing Parts of the Body

The roots used for discussing parts of the body will entail you working with the Latin root in most cases. However, there is always the potential that the roots will come from the Greek. The root that is utilized may be chosen based on how easy it is for a new medical term to be established in the writing process. In addition, these root words may be prepared with combining forms, although not all of these roots will require such forms.

Body Part	Greek Root	Latin Root
abdomen	lapar	abdomen
aorta	aort	aort
arm	brachi	
armpit	maschal	axill
artery	arteri	
back	not	dors
bladder	cyst	vesic
blood (red)	hemat or haemat	sangui
blood clot	thromb	
blood vessel	angi	vascul
bone	oste	ossi

bone marrow	myel	medull
brain	encephala	cerebr
breast	mast	mammo
chest	steth	pector
cheek	parei	bucc
ear	ot	aur
eggs or ova	oo	ov
eye	ophthalm	ocul (may also be optic in French)
eyelid	bluephar	palpebr
face	prosopo	faci
fatty tissues	lip	adip
finger	dactyl	digit
forehead		front
gallbladder	cholecyst	fell
genitalia	phall	
gland	adeno	
glans	balan	
hair	trich	capill
hand	chir	manu
head	cephalo	capito
heart	cardio	cordi
hip		cox
intestine	enter	
jaw	gnath	
kidney	nephr	ren

knee	gon	genu
lip	cheil	labi
liver	hepat	jecor
loin	episi	pudenda
lungs	pneumon	pulmon
marrow	myel	medull
mouth	stomat	or
muscle	my	
nail	onych	ungui
navel	omphal	umbilic
neck	trachel	cervic
nerve	neur	nerv
nose	rhin	nas
ovary	oophor	ovari
pelvis	pyel	pelv
penis	pe	
pupil	cor	
rib	pleur	cost
rib cage	thorac	
shoulder	om	humer
sinus		sinus
skin	dermat	cut
skull	crani	
stomach	gastr	ventr
testis	orchid	

throat (upper)	pharyng	
throat (lower)	laryng	
tooth	odont	dent
tongue	glott	lingu
toe	dactyl	digit
tumor	onc	tum
ureter	ureter	ureter
urethra	urethr	urethr
urinary system	ur	urin
uterus	hyster	uter
vagina	colp	vagin
vein	phleb	ven
vulva	episi	vulv
wrist	carp	carp

Describing Concerns

Some root words may describe physical issues that the body might experience. These include concerns that relate to the body's natural functions. These root words can be used as prefixes in some cases, although they may appear immediately before a suffix as well. These root words may also be part of words that are paired with another word that includes a different root word focusing on the body part that is being influenced or discussed.

Root Word	Greek Root	Latin Root
bent	ankyl	prav
big	mega	magn
broad	eury	lat
cold	cryo	frigi

correctional	ortho	recti
dead	necro	mort
equal	iso	equi
false	pseudo	fals
fast	tachy	celer
feminine	thely	
flat	platy	plan
good	eu	ben
great	mega, megalo	magni
hard	sclera	duri
heavy	bar	grav
hollow	coelo	cavi
improper	dys	mal, mis
irregular	poikil	
larger	megist	maxim
long	macro	longi
male	arseno	vir
narrow	steno	angust
new	neo	novi
normal	ortho	recti
old	paleo	veter
sharp	oxy	ac
short	brachy	brevi
small	micro	parv, minim
slow	brady	tard

soft	malac	moll
straight	ortho	recti
thick	pachy	crass
variable		vari
wide-ranging	eury	lati

Combining Forms

There are times when there is an extra letter at the end of one of these root words. The letter will produce a combining form. The letter allows the two separate words to be joined together.

The word "hematocrit" is a good example of this. "Hemat" is a root word for blood. "Crit" is a suffix that refers to something being separate. The hematocrit will refer to the volume of red blood cells versus the entire volume of blood. The "o" in the middle is required to allow the two parts to link to each other. "Hematocrit" is then easier to read and understand.

There may be cases where multiple parts of the word may be combined without having to add the combining letter. For instance, the word "cystitis" refers to an infection or inflammation in the bladder with "cyst" being the root word and "itis" referring to the suffix. There is no need to add a combining letter.

There are three rules to consider:

1. A vowel will appear in between the root and the suffix. This may include a vowel that is already in either part, although a connecting vowel may be included.

"Rhinitis" is inflammation of the nose and does not need an extra connecting vowel.

2. A combining letter is used when a suffix starts with a consonant.

"Rhinoplasty" refers to the reconstruction of the nose tissue and needs the "o" to connect the two parts. The "o" is the combining letter.

3. A combining letter links one root word to a second root word. This would form a compound word. It doesn't matter if the second root word starts up with a vowel.

For example, "bronchopathy" is a condition relating to air passages within the lungs. The two root words are connected with an "o".

Chapter 18 – Suffixes

Suffixes may be used following terms relating to various parts of the human body. The main purposes for suffixes are to identify a particular condition, a test that may be conducted, or a procedure that may be conducted.

Recognizing the end of the word as it is spoken to you should help you quickly identify what is being referred to.

General Suffixes

The following suffixes are among the more common ones that may be found in various words. For instance, "cardiac" means "relating to the heart," as the suffix "ac" means relating to and "cardi" is the heart.

Suffix	Meaning
ac	relating to
al	relating to
ary	involving
crine	to secrete something
desis	binding
form	having the form of something
gen	coming from something or being of a certain kind
genic	relating to the production of something
gnosis	knowledge, including an identified process
ium	a structure or type of tissue
oid	resembling
osis	increase in something
version	turning

For example, "neurogenic" means "relating to the production of tissues in the nervous system." The suffix "genic" indicates that this is a concept relating to the the root word "neuro."

Identifying Parts of the Body or Activities Within the Body

These suffixes indicate how a condition relates to a body or other action.

Suffix	Meaning
dactyl	relating to a finger or toe
esophageal	involving the esophagus
geusia	the ability or sense of taste
poiesis	when something is produced
ptysis	spitting, or a process where a tissue is spewing
rrhage	when something bursts forward in the body
spadias	an opening in the body; this may be a natural opening or a condition that develops due to an ailment
stalsis	the contraction of a tissue or muscle
stasis	when something stops in the body
staxis	a material dripping out of the body
trophy	the general development or nourishment of the body; this may be the body not receiving the proper nourishment depending on the prefix or root used
vory	about eating

For example, "hematopoiesis" is a process where blood is produced in the body.

Medical Treatments

These suffixes involve some of the medical treatments that may be provided to patients. These include compounds that will target specific areas in the body.

Suffix	Meaning
ase	an enzyme produced within the body
cidal	a compound that kills or destroys something
cide	a material used for eliminating certain compounds in the body

| tion | a reaction that takes place within the body, or a treatment designed to trigger a specific reaction |

Identifying Physical Problems

The following suffixes may be combined with root words to identify the specific physical problem that a person has and where the condition may be located.

Suffix	Meaning
algia	pain
asis	the presence of something
asthenia	weakness
cele	hernia
dipsia	thirst
dynia	involving pain
ectasia	the expansion or enlargement of a tissue or body part
emesis	vomiting
emia	condition relating to blood
iasis	the presence of something; the i may be needed depending on the original word
icle	small in size, or when something shrinks in size
ism	a disease or specific condition
ismus	a spasm or involuntary movement
itis	inflammation
lepsis	an attack or other harmful event
lepsy	a seizure; this may be an actual seizure in the brain or another brain event that triggers sudden changes in one's behaviors or physical functions
lysis	the separation or destruction of something

malacia	when a tissue starts to soften; this includes a tissue that may be harder than others
megaly	when something becomes enlarged
oma	a tumor or collection of mass; this may refer to benign and malignant tumors
omata	the plural form of tumors
osis	condition that does not include inflammation
paresis	a slight form of paralysis; this does not include the total shutdown of a part of the body
pathy	about a disease
ped	involving the foot
penia	a deficiency of a certain compound or nutrient
pepsia	relating to digestion
pes	surrounding a foot
pexy	a fixation on something
phagia	about eating
philia	having an attraction for; this includes a condition that has an attraction and impacts a certain part of the body or another system
phobia	a fear; this may entail something that is minimal, thus leading to a person becoming worried about something minimal in nature
plasia	the formation of a condition; this includes the evolved development of the issue
plegia	paralysis; this includes the complete loss of functionality
plexy	seizure or stroke
ptosis	a prolapse, or the falling or drooping of a tissue
rrhagia	a sudden flow of blood; this includes blood moving quickly in one tissue

rrhea	the flowing of something; this includes items flowing out of a part of the body or a discharge developing
rrhexis	rupture of a tissue
rrhoea	an alternate form of –rrhea, referring to the flowing or discharging of something
rupt	when something breaks or bursts
sclerosis	when a tissue hardens
stenosis	when a structure narrows; the term usually refers to blood vessels but may also be about other parts of the body
tension	pressure
tensive	when a material produces pressure followed by certain concerns
tony	tension in part of the body
tripsy	a crushing feeling in the body

For example, "adenostenosis," refers to a blood vessel narrowing. The suffix "stenosis" infers the idea of the condition developing.

Testing Terms

Testing terms identify cases that uses a particular tool. A prefix may also be used at the beginning of that word to identify where on the body the testing will be conducted.

Suffix	Meaning
gram	picture, or the process of taking a picture
graph/graphy	taking a picture
meter	a tool that measures the count of something; this may also be a function that takes place in the body
metry	a process of measuring something
opsy	an examination or inspection; this may be removing a tissue from the body such as in a biopsy
scope	an instrument that views things inside the body

scopy	the use of an instrument for viewing
tome	a cutting instrument
tomy	the cutting with a surgical instrument

For example, "endoscope" is a tool that will enter into a hollow cavity in the body. This has the prefix "endo" for something being inside of or within the body. A "cardioscope" would involve an instrument that reviews areas inside the heart tissue.

Procedural Terms

These terms refer to the physical treatments that may be provided to a patient to relieve certain conditions. These may be paired with root words to identify the specific part of the body that is to receive a procedure.

Suffix	Meaning
ation	a general process
centesis	surgical opening required for aspiration
ectomy	removal of a mass or part
otomy	the process of making a cut in the body; this may include a partial removal
plasty	the modification of a part of the body or repair; also known as plastic surgery
rrhaphy	a surgical procedure where a suture will be applied
stomy	producing an opening in the body

An example is the word "rhinoplasty." The condition refers to the modification of the nose. This may also be the operation of plastic surgery of the nose.

Specialists

A specialist is a person who is dedicated to a certain field of study that involves a specific segment of the body.

Suffix	Meaning
iatry	medical treatment field

iatrist	a specialist who offers services in a certain field
ics	a field of knowledge or a line of treatment
ist	a person who specializes in reviewing or treating a certain body part or disease
ologist	also a professional who cares for a person or condition
ology	the study of a part of the body; an o may not be necessary depending on the root word
or	a person who will perform a certain medical task

Directional Terms

Directional prefixes and suffixes are used when analyzing the positions of parts of the body, the ways certain bodily functions are operating, and how a procedure is to take place.

Prefix or Suffix	Meaning
ab	away from or the opposite direction of
ad	toward or in the direction of
epi	above
infra	below
inter	within
per	throughout
sub	underneath
ward	in the direction of
wise	directionally

Basic Suffixes

The suffixes listed here refer to some of the more common considerations. These suffixes focus on different meanings.

Suffix	Meaning
able	can be
ed	past tense; this may be added to a verb or adjective
en	made of
er	a person who or someone who is connected to a certain activity; this may be found added to nouns or verbs
er	more of something; this refers to adjectives
est	the most in something; this may be in a comparison of many items with one adjective being used
ful	full of; this occurs after a noun
ial	having characteristics of
ible	is able to be
ic	having certain behaviors
ing	engaging in an activity; this is for a present participle
ion	the act or process of something; the suffix may be preceded by a t, at, or ti
ite	resembling something
ity	a state of; the i is not needed if the last letter is a vowel
ive	an adjective form of a noun; at or it may appear at the start depending on the word
less	without; following a noun or idea
ly	how something could be
ment	the state of being or an act of being something
ness	a state or condition of
or	a person who is linked to an event
ous	having the qualities of; e or I may appear beforehand depending on the word and what fits the best

s	more than one; an 'es' may be necessary if the original noun ends in a consonant
tic	relating to
ula	small
ule	minimal
y	characterized by

Chapter 19 – Building Medical Terms

To identify medical terms, there are three important steps:

1. The suffix of the term.

The suffix is always the first part of the word to review. The suffix should give you a clear idea of the type of effort being handled. This includes a look at the procedure to complete, the test that will take place, or anything else involved.

2. The first part of the word.

You will come across either a root word or the prefix to identify the part of the body that needs to be treated or the kind of issue that might develop.

3. The middle part of the word.

Sometimes a word will only include two parts. However, in other cases, a word may include the root or a connecting letter that links the root to the suffix.

For instance, you might come across a word to explain the inflammation of a person's kidney. The suffix "itis" emphasizes that the condition is inflammation. "Nephr" is the root word for kidney. Combined, the word would be "nephritis."

Another example is the word "hypercalcemia." The definition of this word can be determined by analyzing the three parts. First, "emia" suggests that the condition is in the blood. The "hyper" prefix indicates the condition is greater than usual. "Calc" in the middle refers to the development of calcium in the body. The three parts will combine to form "hypercalcemia," a condition where the blood has excess calcium.

Chapter 20 – Plural Forms

A plural term indicates there is two or more of something. However, you cannot assume that the letter "s" or the letters "es" will appear at the end of a term in its plural form. The last few letters of a term indicate the plural form.

For instance, you may see the word "thorax." The proper plural form for the word is "thoraces" - remove the "x" and replace it with "ces" to create the plural.

The following chart is the specific letters that indicate the plural forms of singular words. These relate to how you'll replace a letter at the end of a word with another letter or a series of letters. This is also for instances where the letter "s" or "es" cannot be easily added to the end of a singular word.

Singular Ending	Plural Ending
a	e
ex	ices
is	es
itis	itides
ix	ices
nx	nges
on	a
um	a
us	i
x	ces
y	ies

These plural replacements are the endings of singular words. For instance, "ovary" would become "ovaries" and "larynx" would become "larynges."

Chapter 21 – Greek vs. Latin

You may find some terms that are written in either the Greek or Latin form. The two languages are different from one another and can directly influence the medical terms that are used. These languages have been used over the years and are the origins of many English words especially in medicine and science terminology.

Throughout this guide, some Greek and Latin terms may be used in the suffixes, prefixes, and root words in medicine.

Greek

The Greek language is from the Hellenic branch of the Indo-European family of languages. The language is the one that is used in Greece and Cyprus. The language is considered a living language because it is actively used, thus making it different from Latin as it is not a living language.

The Greek language is a verb-subject-object language. In this case, the sentences have their critical terms arranged in that order. When it comes to word structure, the Greek terms have the quality of the condition being listed at the start as part of the prefix. The subject in the word will appear in the middle part as the root word.

An important aspect of Greek terms is that the letters are different from what is used in the traditional Greek language. The letters used in the Greek terms are loosely based on the sounds that are produced by the original letters in the Greek alphabet and not the letters themselves.

Latin

The other language that many of the medical terms Latin. While the Greek language is active and used today, the Latin language is no longer used in society. Still, the terms that originated from the language are necessary to know.

The Latin language was prominent in the Middle Ages. This is a language that had been used by the Romans. This belongs in the Italic branch of the Indo-European family of languages. The language is considered to have been vital in the development of various Romance languages including French, Spanish, Italian, and Portuguese.

Latin is often used to introduce concepts relating to the body and its functions. You will recognize Latin in many prefixes and root words.

Should You Study These Languages?

It is not necessary to study these languages to understand the terms that you will encounter your medical work. However, it is critical for you to know the root words.

Chapter 22 – Antonyms

There are often times when you will be presented with antonyms. These antonyms often have one or two letters that are different from one another.

Antonyms are generally made by adding a prefix to the root word which changes the meaning to be opposite. They are easy to confuse.

Prefixes	Meanings
Ab	Moving from an area
Ad	Moving away from an area
Endo	Inside
Exo	Outside
Pre	Before
Post	After
Proximal	Near
Distal	Away
Inferior	Below
Superior	Above
Eu	Regular and positive
Dys	Irregular and negative
Hyper	More than
Hypo	Less than

Retro	Backward
Antero	Forward
Bio	Life
Necro	Death
Tachy	Fast
Brady	Slow
Cepha	Upward
Caudo	Downward
Melano	Black
Leuko	White

Refer to the segment on prefixes for additional examples.

Chapter 23 – Homonyms

Homonyms are words that have the same pronunciation but the words have separate meanings. While you can identify the differences between these words in a written sense, there is a potential that you may hear these words aurally and confuse one for the other.

The following chapter includes a series of homonyms that you may encounter. These words are pronounced alike or similar but have radically different meanings.

Anuresis	An inability to pass urine
Enuresis	Uncontrolled urination, particularly at night
Apophysis	A portion of the bone that is sticking out
Epiphysis	A rounded edge of a bone
Aural	Relating to the ear
Oral	Relating to the mouth
Cor	Involving the heart
Core	The midway part of a measurement or mass
Dyskaryosis	A change in a cell that may be a predictor of a malignant cancer
Dyskeratosis	The hardening of proteins in the hair and skin
Dysphagia	Difficulty with swallowing
Dysphasis	An inability to comprehend speech due to injury or disease
Galactorrhea	An unusual case of milk flowing from the breasts at an excess rate

Galacturia	When the urine develops a milky look to it
Humeral	Relating to the humerus bone
Humoral	Relating to body fluids
Hypothysis	Relating to the pituitary gland
Hypothesis	An analysis of a condition with the goal of finding a possible explanation
Ileum	A portion of the small intestine between the cecum and jejunum
Ilium	A large portion of the pelvic bone
Lice	Small parasites that may impact hair
Lyse	To destroy
Malleous	A bone-like projection in the ankle with a mallet-like look
Malleus	A bone in the middle ear that also has a mallet-like look
Metaphysis	The long part on the top end of a longer bone
Metastasis	When a malignant growth develops outside of the area cancer originated in
Mucous	A membrane or another body that secretes mucus
Mucus	A secretion that is produced by the mucous membrane; the fluid assists in protecting parts of the body

Osteal	A condition involving the bones
Ostial	A concern over an opening in a surgical procedure
Profuse	An issue that is persistent and is excessive
Perfuse	To allow some fluid within the tissue to flow accordingly
Radicle	A small segment in a nerve
Radical	A general effort in a treatment designed to attempt to clear out every aspect of the disease that one has
Resection	When a part of an organ or another segment of the body is removed
Recession	A surgical procedure in the eye to assist in aligning the eyes correctly
Tract	The passageway that oxygen, fluids, or other items may move through; this can include the respiratory or urinary tract
Track	The route at which an injection is to be administered
Vesicle	A small sac that carries fluids
Vesical	A concern that relates to the bladder
Viscus	An internal organ
Viscous	Flows slowly out of the body; this may be used to describe when a secretion takes place in the body

Chapter 24 – Abbreviations and Acronyms

In many cases, time is of the essence when it comes to taking care of patients. As a result, people often use abbreviations when referring to certain conditions.

Abbreviations may be used to keep some things that are on labels less complicated. This is especially when writing prescriptions. By using abbreviations, it becomes easier for people to identify the concepts or considerations in a report.

Also, abbreviations may work in cases where a condition or concept might be quite difficult to write out. Some words or ideas might be easy to misspell.

Acronyms may be used when there are multiple words in a report that has to be summarized.

The following chapter mentions the most commonly used abbreviations in the medical field. These may be used in official reports and in other messages that may be sent to professionals, such as text messages and Twitter messages.

Notes: Some of the abbreviations you will encounter are written in upper-case letters, while others use lower-case. These abbreviations may have radically different meanings. For example, PO means post-operative, while po means that something is to be taken per os or by mouth.

Some abbreviations may have multiple meanings. For example, PVC stands for the premature ventricular complex or for polyvinyl chlorine.

Medical Conditions

Medical abbreviations are mainly acronyms used to shorten the expression. Refer to the chapters surrounding individual body systems throughout this guide for confirmation of the explanations of these medical conditions.

ABG	arterial blood gas; this may also refer to a test used to identify the acidic or oxygen and carbon dioxide levels of blood in the patient's body
ACLS	advanced cardiac life support
AF	atrial fibrillation
AIDS	acquired immunodeficiency syndrome
AMI	acute myocardial infraction
AMS	altered mental status; the condition may be either a person experiencing a condition before treatment or the effects of a treatment

AP	angina pectoris
ARDS	adult respiratory distress syndrome
ASHD	arteriosclerotic heart disease
CA	cardiac arrest
CA	cancer; further details on the type of cancer may be specified by listing a body part, organ, or other abbreviation relating to another part of the body
CAD	coronary artery disease
CHF	congestive heart failure
COLD	chronic obstructive lung disease
COPD	chronic obstructive pulmonary disease
CP	chest pain; this may be a general issue
CP	cerebral palsy
CSM	carotid sinus massage
CSM	cerebrospinal meningitis
CVA	cerebrovascular accident
DM	diabetes mellitus
DOE	dyspnea on exertion; the issue may develop even if the patient is not having a difficulty breathing. The person may experience dyspnea when performing activities.
DTs	delirium tremens
DVT	deep vein thrombosis
fx	fracture; details on where the fracture is must be added
GSW	gunshot wound; additional info is required on the location of the wound and any effects following the incident
H/A	headache
HH	hiatal hernia
HIV	human immunodeficiency virus

HTN	hypertension; specific blood pressure numbers may be laid out next to the listing
IDDM	insulin-dependent diabetes mellitus
IPPB	intermittent positive pressure breathing
JVD	jugular venous distention
LE	lupus erythematosus
LOC	loss of consciousness; this includes LOC situations before, during, or after the treatment process
LOC	level of consciousness; this may be used when analyzing response to a treatment
LR	lactated Ringer's
MAE	moves all extremities; the report may work in the event of significant injury or if there is suspected damage to the central nervous system
MAEW	moves all extremities well; this may include a limitation in how some extremities are capable of working
MI	myocardial infarction
MS	multiple sclerosis
MVA	motor vehicle accident; injuries in such a situation may not be significant
MVC	motor vehicle crash; injuries are more likely to be intense in the situation
NAD	no apparent distress; the patient may not express any particular diseases but needs to be examined for confirmation
NIDDM	non-insulin-dependent diabetes mellitus
NKA	no known allergies; further testing may be required to determine what is causing an allergic reaction or another distress-related event
NKDA	no known drug allergies; this may be used in cases where a patient is to be treated with drugs or in instances where the patient's body might respond differently to certain treatments
N/V	nausea and vomiting; both concerns may not develop at the same time

N/V/D	nausea, vomiting, and diarrhea; this may be listed when the patient experiences all of these concerns
NVD	neck vein distention
OBS	organic brain syndrome
OD	overdose
Pe	pulmonary embolism
PEA	pulseless electrical activity
PEARL	pupils equal and reactive to light; the pupils are capable of responding to any tests that are completed
PERL	pupils equal and reactive to light; this is the same meaning as above
PERRL	pupils equal, round, and reactive to light
PID	pelvic inflammatory disease
PND	paroxysmal nocturnal dyspnea
PSVT	paroxysmal supraventricular tachycardia
PTA	plasma thromboplastin antecedent
PVD	peripheral vascular disease
RA	rheumatoid arthritis
RAD	reactive airway disease
RAD	right axis deviation
RHD	rheumatic heart disease
RL	Ringer's lactate
ROM	rupture of membranes; the concern may develop around any part of the body
SIDS	sudden infant death syndrome
SOB	shortness of breath

STD	sexually transmitted disease; not all reports will go into detail on the STD that is listed. This is to ensure the protection of the patient's identity and, in many cases, out of respect for the patient.
SVT	supraventricular tachycardia
TB	tuberculosis
TIA	transient ischemic attack
URI	upper respiratory infection; this may be whooping cough, effects of a cold or flu, laryngitis, or another issue that impacts the upper respiratory system
VD	venereal disease; this may be another sexually transmitted disease, but it could be any other situation. Again, this may require privacy over the details surrounding the disease and how sensitive the condition is.

Physical Body Parts or Functions

The following listing includes body parts and various aspects inside the body that require treatment needs.

abd	abdomen
a/g	a measure of the ratio of albumin in the blood versus globulin
AK	above the knee; this may entail anything above that area
A-line	arterial line
ant	anterior
AP	anteroposterior or front-to-back
AP	anterior pituitary
AP	arterial pressure
APC	atrial premature complex
BBB	bundle branch block
BK	below the knee; this can include any segment under the knee
BM	bowel movement
BP	blood pressure

BS	blood sugar
BS	breath sounds; this includes an analysis of how normal certain concerns are
BSA	body surface area
CA	coronary artery
CBC	complete blood count
C&S	culture sensitivity test; used to determine the possible pathogen in the body in order to determine the proper treatment for a condition
CSF	cerebrospinal fluid
CVP	central venous pressure
DTR	deep tendon reflexes; these may be determined based on how well the patient responds to a reflex test, such as when a doctor hits a patient's tendon with a hammer-like instrument
ENT	ears, nose, and throat; this can also refer to a condition that relates to one of these areas
ET	endotracheal area; this includes an area that is within the trachea
FBS	fasting blood sugar
FHR	fetal heart rate
FHT	fetal heart tones
FSH	follicle-stimulating hormone
GB	gallbladder
GI	gastrointestinal; this includes parts of the GI system and any conditions or events that might influence the GI system
GU	genitourinary
gyn	gynecology
H&H	hemoglobin and hematocrit levels in the blood
Hb	hemoglobin apart from other blood contents
Hct	hematocrit separate from other bodies

Hgb	hemoglobin
I&O	intake and output referring to how much is consumed at a time
IC	inspiratory capacity referring to how well the body handles air
ICP	intracranial pressure
IC	irritable colon
IM	intramuscular
IO	intraosseous
KUB	kidneys, ureters, and bladder; this is for cases where the condition has spread to all of these parts of the body
LE	left eye
LE	lower extremity
LLL	left lower lobe in the lung
LLQ	left lower quadrant in the abdomen
LUL	left upper lobe in the lug
LUQ	left upper quadrant in the abdomen
NPA	nasopharyngeal airway
NSR	normal sinus rhythm
O2	oxygen
OD	right eye
OPA	oropharyngeal airway
OS	left eye
OU	both eyes; this is for cases where a condition has impacted both eyes or for when a drug has to be administered in both eyes
PEEP	positive end-expiratory pressure
pH	hydrogen ion concentration; this may be found in the blood or other parts of the body

PO2	partial oxygen pressure
PVC	premature ventricular complex
RA	right atrium of the heart
RBC	red blood cell
Rh	Rhesus blood factor
Rh	rhodium
RLL	right lower lobe in the lung
RLQ	right lower quadrant of the abdomen
ROM	range of motion; this refers to how well a person can move certain body parts with ease
RUL	right upper lobe of the lung
RUQ	right upper quadrant of the abdomen
SC	subcutaneous
SC	secretory component or segment of the body where a secretion may be based
SL	sublingual
SubQ	subcutaneous; this refers to the part of the skin
SQ	subcutaneous, for the skin
TPR	temperature, pulse, and respiration; all three may be listed at once in the same report
UA	urinalysis
UE	upper extremity
VS	vital signs; these may be a pulse, breathing, and other indications that prove a person is alive
WBC	white blood cell

Care Instructions

The abbreviations in this segment refer to both the processes that may be used or any measurements that are needed for the treatment process.

ä	before
ää	of each (used when writing a prescription)
ac	before a meal; this is mainly in reference to when someone is to take a medication
ad-lib	as much as needed
amb	ambulatory; this refers to activities relating to walking
AMA	against medical advice; this would be for cases where a patient demands a certain procedure or routine even if a doctor has suggested that it may be too risky or dangerous
AED	Automated external defibrillator
AKA	above the knee amputation
AOx4	alert issues to person, place, self, and time
APC	activated protein C
Ag	water
ASA	aspirin or acetylsalicylic acid
ASAP	as soon as possible
AV	arteriovenous (as in administration)
bid	to be completed twice a day; this does not include specific hours in the day
BKA	below the knee amputation
bx	biopsy
ć	with
Ca	calcium
CABG	coronary artery bypass graft
cap	capsule, referring to the way a drug may be administered

cc	cubic centimeter
CC	chief complaint; this may be the greatest concern for the patient. The complaint should be the reason why the person is asking for help.
CCU	coronary care unit
Cl	chloride
cm	centimeter
cm3	cubic centimeter
c/o	complaining of; this may not be the chief complaint in all cases. This could be a person complaining of a certain effect of a treatment.
CO	carbon monoxide
CO	the patient's cardiac output
CO2	carbon dioxide
CPR	cardiopulmonary resuscitation
CRNA	certified registered nurse anesthetist
CRT	capillary refill time
CRT	cathode ray tube
CSF	cerebrospinal fluid
CXR	chest x-ray
D&C	dilation and curettage
D/C	discontinue the process; this may be based on certain medical standards or by the patient's request for treatment
diff	differential
dig	digoxin
DNR	do not resuscitate; in this case, the patient does not request any particular efforts from medical professionals to resuscitate him/her in the event of an emergency. This may be written for those who are near death and want to die peacefully.
DOA	dead on arrival

DON	Director of nursing
DOS	dead on scene
DPT	diphtheria, pertussis, and tetanus vaccine
DSD	dry sterile dressing
DtaP	diphtheria, tetanus, and acellular pertussis vaccine
DTP	diphtheria, tetanus, and pertussis vaccine
D5W	dextrose 5 percent in water
Dx	diagnosis
ECG	electrocardiogram
ED	emergency department
EDC	estimate date of confinement; this may be the start of treatment
EEG	electroencephalogram
eg	for example
EKG	electrocardiogram
ER	emergency room
ET	endotracheal tube; this may be used to administer treatments
ETA	Estimated time of arrival; this would be when the patient was brought into a medical facility for treatment and especially for emergency treatment
ETOH	ethyl alcohol
ETT	endotracheal tube
F1O2	fraction of inspired oxygen for treatment needs
Fe	iron
FHx	family history
fL	femtoliter
fl	fluid
fld	fluid

g	gram
gm	gram
gr	grain
gtt	drop; this may be used when administering intravenous drugs
GTT	glucose tolerance test
h	hour
H	hypodermic; this focuses mainly on injections and treatments
H&P	history and physical data
Hg	mercury; this may be used mainly to refer to blood pressure tests
H2O	water
H2O2	hydrogen peroxide
HPI	history of present illness
hr	hour
hs	at bedtime; this is for procedures or administrations that are to be handled before a person goes to sleep in a treatment facility
Hx	history; this includes a general analysis
ICU	intensive care unit
IM	intramuscular, primarily for how a drug is to be administered through an injection
in vitro	inside the laboratory; this may include a case where the body is impacted by something that is applied within a lab
in vivo	inside the body
IUD	intrauterine device used for contraception
IV	intravenous
K	potassium
KCl	potassium chloride

kg	kilogram
KVO	keep vein open
L	liter
LAC	laceration
LAC	laparoscopic-assisted colectomy
lb	pound
L/m	liters per minute
LMP	last menstrual period
LPM	liters per minute
LPN	licensed practical nurse
LSD	lysergic acid diethylamide
LVN	licensed vocational nurse
m	meter
MAP	mean arterial pressure
mcg	microgram
MCL	modified chest lead
mEq	milliequivalent; this may be an equivalent for how some medications may be used for treatment
mg	milligram; some doctors may use mgm as an abbreviation for clarification or formality
MICU	mobile or medical intensive care unit
min	minute; this refers to the measurement of time
mL	milliliter
mm	millimeter
mm Hg	millimeters of mercury; this may be used for pressure-related tests including for blood pressure testing

MRI	magnetic resonance imaging
MS	morphine sulfate
MSO4	morphine sulfate
n	normal, referring to conditions not changing beyond usual
Na	sodium
NA	not applicable
NaCl	sodium chloride
NaHCO3	sodium bicarbonate
NC	nasal cannula; this refers to a material that is inserted into the nasal passage during a procedure
NG	nasogastric
NICU	neonatal intensive care unit; the system is designed for the treatment of children and newborns who have certain medical concerns
NPO	nil per os; nothing by mouth, or the patient is not allowed to consume anything orally
NTG	nitroglycerin
OD	outside diameter
OP	outpatient; this refers to when a patient requires medical services and does not have to stay in the hospital for an extended period
OR	operating room
oz	ounce
p	after, including following a procedure or when someone is to take a medication
pc	after meals; this may include every meal of the day and can indicate when a medication is to be taken
PCO2	partial pressure of carbon dioxide

PDR	Physicians' Desk Reference; this book lists information on medications and how they are to be administered. The book is updated every year and is found in most medical treatment facilities.
ped	pediatric or relating to treating a child's condition
po	per os, to be administered by mouth
PO	postoperative procedure or post-op
PR	per rectum; this is for when a suppository is to be administered in the rectal cavity
PRN	pro re nata; this indicates a medication or process is to be completed as needed
psi	pounds per square inch; this may be used in blood pressure tests
pt	patient
PT	physical therapy
PTA	prior to admission, or events that took place before the patient reached a treatment facility
PVC	polyvinyl chloride
q	every; this is the basis for instructions on how often a person is to take a medication or any other type of intervention that must take place
q12	every twelve hours; a different number may be listed to specify the exact number of hours when something has to be done.
qAM	every morning
qd	every day
qh	every hour
qhs	before bedtime
qid	four times in a day
qod	every other day
qPM	every evening
RN	registered nurse

R/O	rule out; in this case, you can rule out certain physical treatments that might not be as effective as hoped
Rx	prescription
ŝ	without
SICU	surgical intensive care unit
ss	half
S/S	signs and symptoms
stat	immediately
Sx	symptoms
sym	symptoms
T	temperature as measured by a thermometer; this may be followed with a C or F depending on whether the Celsius or Fahrenheit is used
tab	tablet, as in a drug for administration
TBA	to be admitted
TBA	to be announced; details on when the announcement can be made could be included provided those details are known
tbsp.	tablespoon
tech	technician or another person to handle technical devices or functions in the work environment
tid	three times a day
TKO	to keep open; this may be a surgical opening or another area that has to be secured
tsp	teaspoon
Tx	treatment
U	unit
vol	volume, usually of a liquid treatment
w/	with

WNL	within normal limits; a recommendation for how a patient is to be treated
w/o	without
wt	weight
yo	years old
x	except
1	first degree or primary
2	second degree or secondary; this may be an effect of a condition that goes alongside the primary concern

Specialty Symbols

The following symbols are often used in the treatment process to refer to very specific instructions. These are not always used in medical reports, but they may help identify what has to be done when taking care of a patient.

↑	increase; this is for elevated symptoms or to increase the dosage
↓	decrease; for when symptoms decline or to reduce the dosage
1o	first degree
2o	second degree
3o	third degree
θ	none
(R)	right
(L)	left
μ	micro
α	alpha
β	beta
~	approximate
x2	doubled or times two
/	per

≠	not equal to
>	greater than
<	less than
?	possible or questionable
-	negative
♂	male
♀	female

Such symbols may be used to save time when writing notes surrounding certain conditions or treatments that have to be followed.

Pharmacy Abbreviations

The following listing of abbreviations focuses on things that you may notice in prescriptions. These abbreviations are produced by doctors who prescribe medications to patients to clarify how something is to be administered. The terms are also included to save room on the label for a drug to ensure more information can be included.

Note: Some of the abbreviations are derived from Latin terms. The Latin terms, if applicable, are listed in parentheses next to the meaning in question.

aa	each (ana)
AAA	apply to the affect area
ac	before a meal (ante cibum)
ad	right ear (auris dextra)
ad lib	as much as needed (ad libitum, at one's desire)
am	morning or before noon (ante meridiem)
amp	ampule (a glass container used for measuring the total amount of something)
amt	amount
APAP	acetaminophen
aq	water (aqua)
as	left ear (auris sinistra)

ATC	around the clock, or at various points in the day
au	both ears (auris utraque)
bib	drink (bibe)
bid	twice in a day (bis in die)
BP	blood pressure
bucc	inside the cheek (bucca)
c	with (cum)
cc	cubic centimeter
cc	with food (cum cibo; this is not used as often)
cap	capsule
cm	centimeter
cm	cream (for topical application)
d	day
DAW	dispense as written, or to follow the instructions for specific use
dc	discontinue
dil	dilute
disp	dispense
div	divide
dL	deciliter
DR	delayed release
EC	enteric-coated
eod	every other day
er	extended release
et	and (et)
ft	to make (fiat)

fl	fluid
FXD	for 10 days (X refers to the Roman number for 10)
g	gram
gm	gram
gal	gallon
gr	grain
gtt	drop (gutta)
h	hour (hora)
hs	at bedtime (hora somni)
id	intradermal
im	intramuscular
in	intranasal
inf	infusion
inh	inhalation
inj	injection
IR	immediate release
IU	international unit; a form of measuring technical compounds
IV	intravenous
kg	kilogram
L	liter
lb	pound (libra)
liq	liquid
lot	lotion
max	maximum
min	minimum

neb	nebulizer
od	right eye (oculus dexter)
ODT	oral distintegrating tablet
oint	ointment
os	left eye (oculus sinister)
OTC	over the counter
ou	both eyes (oculus uterque)
PA	prior authorization; this includes confirming that a drug can be used
pc	after a meal (post cibum)
pm	evening or after the noon hour (post meridiem)
po	orally or by mouth (per os)
pr	rectally (per rectum)
prn	as needed or as needed for the treatment of something (pro re nata)
pv	vaginally or through the vaginal tissue (per vaginam)
q	every (quaque; a number can be added to indicate the number of hours between doses)
qam	every morning (quaque anti meridiem)
qd	every day (quaque die)
qhs	every day when going to bed (quaque hora somni)
qid	four times a day (quarter in die)
qty	quantity
qpm	every evening (quaque post meridiem)
qs	an appropriate quantity (quantum sufficiat)
Rx	prescription (recipere, or to take something)
s	without (sine)
SC	subcutaneous

sig	label (signa)
SL	sublingually
susp	suspension
syr	syrup
tab	tablet
TAD	take as directed
tid	three times in a day (ter in die)
top	topical
troch	lozenge (trochiscus)
ud	as directed (ut dictum)
ung	ointment (unguentum)
w	with
w/f	with food or a meal
w/o	without taking anything else
xr	extended release

Chapter 25 – Measurement Terms

As you take care of medications, treatments, and other important considerations, you may come across some measurement terms. These terms are designed to help you recognize things like how much of medication has to be used, how long an endoscope might be, or the area that a cut is to be made. However, measurement terms can be extremely confusing and frustrating.

Various units of measurement may be used in the medical field. These units identify different types of activities that may take place depending on what has to be measured. Such measures may be identified in a report to ensure there is knowledge of what is being analyzed or diagnosed as well as how certain administrations are to be applied.

Basic Measurements

foot	12 inches
yard	3 feet
rod	5.5 yards
square foot	144 square inches
cubic foot	1,728 cubic inches

Liquid Measurements

pint	4 gills
quart	2 pints
gallon	4 quarts

Liquid Measures for Apothecary Use

fluid dram	60 minims
fluid ounce	8 fluid drams
pint	16 fluid ounces
quart	2 pints or 32 fluid ounces
gallon	4 quarts or 128 fluid ounces

Circulate Measurements

degree	60 minutes

minute	60 seconds
right angle	90 degrees
straight angle	180 degrees
circle	360 degrees

Measurements For Applying Materials

1 teaspoon	5 milliliters
1 teaspoon	1/8 fluid ounce
1 cup	16 liquid teaspoons
1 cup	8 fluid ounces
1 tablespoon	½ fluid ounce
1 tablespoon	3 teaspoons
1 cup	12 dry tablespoons
1 glass	8 fluid ounces or half a pint

Conversions

Note: While many of these conversions are extremely specific, a small bit of leeway can be used when trying to get these measures ready. The best concept for use is to work with as close of a conversion total as possible to ensure the work in question can be handled accordingly.

1 grain	0.0648 gram
1 cubic meter	35.314 cubic feet
1 cubic inch	16.3872 cubic centimeters
1 cubic foot	0.02832 cubic meters
1 liter	2.1134 pints
1 liter	1.0567 quart
1 fluid ounce	29.573 milliliters
1 quart	946.353 milliliters
1 gallon	3.785 liters

Prefixes For Numbers

Some prefixes may be utilized to specify when something is of a certain number. This means that a number is very large or small in size. The number may be to the power of a certain value. For instance, 10^3 would equal 1,000, as this entails 10 being multiplied three times. 10^6 would equal 1,000,000 as well. Meanwhile, a decimal may entail 1 being divided by 10 a certain number of times. In this case, 10^{-2} would be 0.01.

Here is a look at the prefixes that may be utilized:

Prefix	Number	Symbol
deca	10^1	da
hector	10^2	h
kilo	10^3	k
mega	10^6	M
giga	10^9	G
tera	10^{12}	T
deci	10^{-1}	d
centi	10^{-2}	c
milli	10^{-3}	m
micro	10^{-6}	μ
nano	10^{-9}	n
pico	10^{-12}	p
femto	10^{-15}	f
atto	10^{-18}	a

These prefixes may refer to masses or lengths. The symbol would also be used alongside a letter such as g for masses or m for lengths when used to abbreviate the total being measured. For instance, a kilogram would be 1,000 grams or 1,000 kg. A nanogram would be 10^{-9} ng.

Temperature Measurements

You may encounter measurements for temperatures in either Fahrenheit or Celsius. To measure Fahrenheit temperatures, the Celsius temperature is multiplied by 9/5 and then 32 is added. For instance, 10 Celsius would equal 50 Fahrenheit.

To measure a Celsius temperature, subtract 32 from a Fahrenheit temperature and then multiply by 5/9 or 0.5555. Therefore, 103 Fahrenheit would equal 39.444 Celsius.

Pressure

Pressure measurement is the amount of stress that can be applied in an area. The pressure is measured in pounds per square inch or foot. The measurement is used to review blood pressure totals among other functions surrounding how fluids are moving in the body.

The pressure being analyzed is based on mm Hg or millimeters of mercury. The mm Hg total is a unit of pressure based on the added pressure produced by a column of mercury that is one millimeter high. The measurement can be found in a blood pressure test with a higher number suggesting that the blood is not moving as well as it should be. The pressure should be analyzed carefully and is an indication of what is happening within the patient's body.

Blood Test Measurement

Many of the measurements you will encounter when handling blood involves the volume of the blood in question.

A blood measurement is reviewing the quality of the blood based on a certain total. It can be measured in "per liter" or "per gram." When you look at a measurement of blood cells per milliliter, you will be measuring the total number of blood cells that are in a milliliter-sized sample of blood. For cases where you have larger samples, you would have to take the total and divide it by the number of the measurement points you are working with (for 400 million in 3 mL, divide 400 million by 3 = 133.3 million per mL).

The mmol/L measurement is one of the most prominent blood test measurements. This is a millimole per liter. A mole is an amount that involves s a large number of atoms. A mole is specifically 6×10^{23}. A millimole is one-thousandth of a mole (hence the milli prefix). The mmol/L analysis is used to determine a better estimate of what the blood contains.

There are cases where results may change at various times based on physical activity and the diet one has had. A person who is to have a blood test should fast for a certain period before the test takes place. This is to ensure the test will be more accurate. A patient should also disclose any dietary activities or other actions one has participated in prior to the test.

Chapter 26 – Eponyms

Eponyms are medical terms that are named for people. These are not necessarily people who had these conditions, but rather medical professionals who discovered them or in some cases the places that these conditions were first documented.

The effort in generating the names of these conditions is to improve upon how well people can recall the issue and convey information surrounding the concern with others. In some cases, a condition may be named for a person who had the condition. These cases are known as autoenponyms.

For instance, Down Syndrome is named for John Langdon Down, a physicist who classified the genetic condition.

Amyotrophic lateral sclerosis is often referred to as ALS or Lou Gehrig's Disease as the baseball player is one of the most prominent figures to have developed the condition. Most people did not know much about the condition until Lou Gehrig, a high-profile figure, developed the condition. Another example of a condition named for a person is Valentino's syndrome. The condition is a duodenal ulcer named for Rudolph Valentino, a silent film actor who died from an infection triggered by the condition.

Munchausen syndrome is a condition that involves a person faking a disease, for instance. The disorder is named after Baron Munchausen, a fictional character that was known for telling unusual tall tales. The eponym helps the professional recognize the patient who is clearly exaggerating about a condition and may engage in this behavior many times to gain attention from others.

The eponym helps summarize the condition that a person may have and the symptoms of the conditions. Eponyms often refer to medical illnesses, although they may also relate to particular treatments or surgical procedures that may be required.

Note: Some conditions may only be referred to by the first name of the person who is listed in the eponym. Budd-Chiari Syndrome may be referenced in a report as "Budd."

Diseases

The diseases that are named after other people are relative to unique conditions. You may or may not encounter some of these conditions.

Ackerman's Tumor (ack-ur-minz)

An unusual version of squamous cell carcinoma. The condition is a massive lesion that forms on the body. The carcinoma issue may be seen in those who regularly chew tobacco.

Addison's Disease (ad-i-sinz)

Primary adrenocortical deficiency. This is a condition where the adrenal glands are unable to produce cortisol and aldosterone.

Addisonian Anemia

Pernicious anemia. The antibodies in the blood will attack some intrinsic factors in the blood. It becomes difficult for the body to use vitamin B12 as a result.

Aide's Tonic Pupil

The development of a large pupil. The pupil is unable to constrict when it is exposed to light. The pupil may constrict after a while, but it will take some time to do this. The pupil make take some time to dilate as well.

Albright's Syndrome (awl-brites)

The development of hypocalcemia and elevated parathormone levels in the body's serum. The condition may be noted through some unusual spots and discoloration forming in various areas around the patient's body.

Alport's Syndrome (al-ports)

Hereditary nephritis. The nerves in the kidneys start to wear out potentially leading to end state renal disease.

Alzheimer's (alz-high-murz)

A progressive form of dementia that develops as the brain is unable to handle proper connections.

Andersen's Disease

A disease where the body is unable to properly store glycogen. The condition may be due to metabolic errors in the body. The GBE1 gene will have mutated as the condition develops.

Argyll-Robertson Pupil

When the pupil in the eye shrinks in size. The pupil is unable to respond with the proper light reflex due to the condition.

Arnold-Chiari Malformation (chee-our-ee)

A defect found in the cerebellum. A portion of the cerebellum may descend downward causing pains in the neck area, dizziness, vomiting, and difficulty swallowing.

Barlow Disease

May also be called scurvy. This occurs when a person does not have enough ascorbic acid or vitamin C in the body. A person experiences fatigue and weakness. Gum disease and an increase in bleeding from the skin may also develop.

Barrett's Esophagus

Damages in the mucosal cells in the lower area of the esophagus. The condition occurs when unhealthy cells develop and cause the lining in the esophagus to deteriorate. The concern may result in the development of esophageal cancer.

Bartter Syndrome

A defect in the kidney that causes hypokalemia or a decline in potassium levels in the blood. The condition may also trigger alkalosis or an elevated blood pH level plus hypotension.

Becker's Muscular Dystrophy

A form of muscular dystrophy that is benign. The condition does not cause any changes in the skeletal system or the heart, although the muscles may be negatively influenced by the condition.

Bell's Palsy

Inflammation in the facial nerve in the facial canal located in the middle ear. The condition causes facial paralysis where the person is unable to control muscle movements in one part of the face. The condition typically impacts one side of the face, although in rare cases, it may also occur on both sides.

Berger's Disease

A form of nephropathy. The condition exhibits unusual IgA levels deposited in the kidney. The condition promotes inflammation in the kidney. This may also cause some significant concerns surrounding how the body functions.

Berry Aneurysm

An aneurysm that develops in the cerebral arterial circle in the brain. The aneurysm may be more significant than a standard aneurysm in the brain.

Brown-Sequard Syndrome (se-kwa-rd)

A condition that develops when one half of the spinal cord is damaged. The condition will develop in paralysis on the side of the injury and a loss of sensation on the other side of the injury.

Bruton's Disease

A condition where white blood cells are not formed properly. The cells are unable to divide and move about in the body as necessary. The condition may trigger difficulties in the immune system. This includes causing the body to be more likely to develop immune system concerns. The condition is not related to HIV/AIDS, although it can be a sign of significant problems in how the immune system functions.

Budd-Chiari Syndrome

Damage to the hepatic veins in the liver. The veins that regularly drain the liver will be damaged, thus potentially forming blood clots in the area and enlargement of the liver. The liver may stop functioning properly due to the tissue being expanded in size and is not as active or able to work as it should.

Buerger's Disease (bu-er-gurz)

The inflammation of small arteries in the body. The condition may cause some nerves and arteries to collect into one mass, thus producing intense pain. The condition may lead to gangrene depending on how it progresses.

Burkitt's Lymphoma

An intense form of lymphoma that occurs in children. The condition is more prominent in Africa.

Chagas' Disease (chay-gus)

A parasitic infection that promotes heart failure. The parasite may come from a worm, although it could also be any other item that may enter into the heart tissue and cause significant threats to the region.

Conn's Syndrome

An excessive production of aldosterone in the adrenal glands. The condition can cause hyperplasia and, in some cases, may also trigger the development of tumors.

Creutzfeldt-Jakob Disease (crewtz-felt)

Degeneration in the central nervous system. Proteins known as prions develop in the brain and may result in death due to the cerebral system breaking down.

Crigler-Najjar Syndrome (krig-lur-nah-jur)

Neonatal jaundice. This may be because the liver is not functioning properly. Red blood cells may not form normally.

Crohn's Disease (krones)

The development of inflammation in the bowel. The condition may develop around the anus and can include lesions that persistently develop in the region.

Crouzon Syndrome (crew-zahn)

When the branchial arches are not formed properly. This may be noticed by protruding eyes. The eyes may become dry and could be at risk of experiencing fatigue and distress.

Curling's Ulcer

An ulcer that develops in the gastric area. The region erodes due to a lack of plasma volume. The death of cells around the gastric mucosa will cause intense burns in the area. The issue is associated mainly with significant forms of trauma, including sepsis and burns.

Cushing's Syndrome

Hypercortisolism. The body experiences an excessive amount of cortisol, thus reducing the body's ability to respond to stress.

Cushing's Ulcer

Gastritis that develops with intracranial lesions.

de Quervain's Thyroiditis (kwer-vanes)

Inflammation in the thyroid caused by a virus. The tissue becomes enlarged and tender.

DiGeorge's Syndrome

A condition that develops when a portion of chromosome 22 is removed. People with the condition typically experience congenital heart issues, although hearing loss or learning difficulties may also develop among some patients.

Down's Syndrome

A condition where part of a copy of chromosome 21 is found. Excessive gene will cause intellectual disability and growth delays. This may also include distinct facial features. The lifespan of the person may be limited, although it is unclear as to what may happen in this situation regarding how the person's body may develop while experiencing the condition.

Dressler's Syndrome

Pericarditis that occurs following a myocardial infarction.

Dubin-Johnson Syndrome

Hyperbilirubinemia. The liver becomes damaged and may process bilirubin improperly. The fluid may move into the bile, thus reducing its overall functionality.

Duchenne Muscular Dystrophy

A form of muscular dystrophy that occurs mainly at an early age. Muscle weakness will develop alongside significant skeletal or heart conditions.

Edwards Syndrome

A genetic condition when a copy of chromosome 18 develops. The condition will result in low birth weight and heart defects in children. The condition can also cause significant intellectual disability.

Ehlers-Danlos Syndrome (eh-lurs-dan-louse)

When collagen functions improperly in the body. The condition can cause tissues to become fragile and may also cause joints to not function normally. Also, the skin may extend more than expected. The condition may put a person at an elevated risk of fractures, dislocations, and other disorders that relate to connective tissues.

Ehrlichiosis (err-lick-ee-oh-sis)

A bacterial infection spread by ticks. The infection kills white blood cells.

Eisenmenger's Complex (eye-zin-men-gurz)

The reversal of a left to right shunt. A patient may develop an open path between both sides of the heart, thus producing an inefficient control over the tissue.

Erb's-Duchenne Palsy (urbz-dou-chin)

Paralysis in the arm caused by damages to the nerves in the body. This includes the severing of some nerves in the spinal column.

Ewing Sarcoma

A round cell tumor found in the bone tissue

Fabry's Disease

A disease where lipids deposit in the organs. The organs will eventually fail.

Fanconi's Syndrome

A lack of reabsorption in the kidney.

Felty's Syndrome

The development of rheumatoid arthritis, a lack of neutrophils in the blood, and an enlargement of the spleen.

Gardner's Syndrome

The development of polyps within the colon. This may be paired with osteomas and soft tumors around the tissues.

Gaucher's Disease (go-churz)

The erosion of long bones within the body; this includes the femoral heads of these bones wearing out.

Gilbert's Syndrome

A defect where bilirubin is not processed properly.

Glanzmann's Thrombasthenia (glan-zee-min throm-bas-teen-ee-ah)

A bleeding disorder where the platelets do not contain fibrinogen. The fibrinogen is unable to bridge the platelets together, thus causing the patient to bleed longer than usual.

Goodpasture's Syndrome

An autoimmune disorder where antibodies attack the renal system and lungs resulting in organ failure.

Grave's Disease

Damage to the thyroid gland that triggers hyperthyroidism.

Guillain-Barre Syndrome (gill-ain-bare)

Damage around muscle tissues caused by the immune system as it weakens the peripheral nervous system.

Hand-Schuller-Christian Disease

A condition where bone lesions develop on the skull.

Hashimoto's Thyroiditis

Hypothyroidism caused when the immune system attacks the thyroid gland. The gland may develop inflammation, which will eventually lead to the destruction of the gland.

Henoch-Schonlein Purpura (hen-ock schen-leen)

The development of small bleeding found under the skin followed by pains in the joints and abdomen. The condition may also cause the kidneys to process blood and protein and move them into the patient's urine stores.

Hirschprung's Disease (hur-sh-prungz)

When nerves are missing in the intestine. The condition occurs at birth and may lead to constipation. Some children who develop the issue may experience reduced growth rates.

Hodgkin's Lymphoma

A lymphoma where cancer develops from lymphocytes, a form of a white blood cell.

Horner's Syndrome

Damage to the sympathetic trunk. The condition may cause paralysis in an eyelid and changes in the pupil. A person may also experience reduced sweating in warm conditions.

Huntington's Disease

The destruction of brain cells. The condition may evolve into dementia depending on the progress.

Kaposi's Sarcoma

Cancer that develops in the skin and various organs and can produce lesions that are purple and may be flat. The condition develops mainly among those with HIV and AIDS.

Kartagener's Syndrome

Damages to the cilia in the respiratory tract. The cilia will improperly bind together with one another when the condition is present.

Kawasaki Disease

Inflammation of blood vessels around the body. The condition may exhibit a fever that lasts for several days and is not treated properly through the use of medications.

Klinefelter Syndrome (kline-fel-tur)

The development of two or more X chromosomes in males. The condition causes infertility and small testicles.

Kluver-Bucy Syndrome (klu-vur-bu-see)

The development of lesions in the medial temporal lobe. The condition may cause a person to engage in compulsive eating activities.

Krukenberg Tumor (crew-kun-burg)

A malignant ovary produced due to cancerous cells developing from another primary site. In most cases, the condition develops with the gastrointestinal tract being the first place where the issue occurs. The concern may also develop in some other tissues like the breast.

Laennec's Cirrhosis (lay-in-ics)

The development of cirrhosis caused by excessive alcohol consumption.

Lesche-Nyhan Syndrome (lesh-nee-han)

A deficiency in certain enzymes in the body. The condition may cause an excess uric acid and the body is unable to process the compound properly. Gout and mental deficiencies may develop.

Letterer-Siwe Syndrome (let-tur-rur-sue)

Langerhans cell histiocytosis. A potentially fatal condition that causes skin lesions and ear drainage and may eventually move into the muscles in the patient's body.

Libman-Sacks Disease

Endocarditis caused by things other than bacteria. In most cases, the condition may be related to lupus.

Li-Fraumeni Syndrome (lee-frau-min-e)

A cancer condition that may have many primary sites of cancer that form around the body. The sites will develop throughout the patient's life and may require extensive treatment.

Lou Gehrig's Disease (gar-igz)

Amyotrophic lateral sclerosis or ALS. The condition involves the motor neurons around the brain degenerating. The condition leads to a progressive loss of regular body functions and will eventually lead to death.

Mallory-Weis Syndrome

Bleeding from the esophagus. A laceration will develop in the mucosa in the connection between the stomach and esophagus. The condition may develop due to alcoholism or bulimia among other conditions where a person experiences intense vomiting spells. A laceration may also be called a tear.

Marcus-Gunn Pupil

An eye defect. The swinging of light between the eyes will show that the eyes are developing constriction with excess dilation potentially likely to develop in the most intense cases.

Marfan Syndrome

A genetic condition where the connective tissue does not form properly. The condition will cause a person to develop a tall and thin frame and long extremities. The joints may be excessively flexible. Scoliosis is also likely to develop. A person with Marfan syndrome is at a high risk of a possible aortic aneurysm or from a prolapse of various parts of the body.

McArdle's Disease (mik-ar-dulz)

A metabolic condition. The body is unable to storage glycogen properly.

Meckel's Diverticulum (meck-ulz)

A lethal genetic condition. This may be caused by the central nervous system being improperly formed. Pulmonary hypoplasia may develop in some cases.

Meig's Syndrome

Development of ascites, pleural effusion, and a benign ovarian tumor. All three conditions develop at once, although the condition is relieved when the tumor is removed.

Menetrier's Disease (men-eh-tree-urz)

Hyporpteinemic hypertrophic gastropathy. This is a stomach condition that develops due to intense gastric folds and elevated production of mucous. The body will lose its proteins as the stomach is unable to process these tissues. The acid will not be likely to develop. The cause is uncertain.

Meniere's Disease (men-ee-yerz)

A condition that develops in the inner ear. The issue triggers vertigo and tinnitus. This may also cause a feeling of fullness in the ear. Hearing loss may also develop. The condition may be influenced by intense constrictions in blood vessels around the tissue, although autoimmune reactions may also be a factor.

Menkes Disease (mek-kis)

A genetic disorder. The ATP7A protein needed to transport copper fails. The body cannot absorb the copper is requires resulting in liver and nervous system damage. The body may not grow properly. The condition develops among infants and those who develop the condition likely dying before reaching three years of age.

Monckeberg's Arteriosclerosis (mon-key-burgz)

Excess calcification in the body.

Munchausen Syndrome (mun-chow-sin)

Factitious disorder imposed on the self. A person will attempt to fake an illness, disease, or another form of distress to draw attention or sympathy from others. This may be a person attempting to be hospitalized many times while often attempting to tell unusual tales surrounding their experiences.

Nelson's Syndrome

Adrenal stresses that require the surgical removal of the adrenal glands. This may also be called a form of pituitary adenoma.

Niemann-Pick Syndrome

When the body is unable to support lysosomal compounds.

Ormond's Disease

Retroperitoneal fibrosis. A disease where fibrous tissue develops in the retroperitoneum, an area that keeps the kidneys, aorta, and renal system intact. The condition may trigger kidney failure and deep vein thrombosis.

Osler-Weber-Rendu Syndrome

The development of unusual blood vessels forming in the skin and organs. This is a genetic condition that may trigger excess nosebleeds, bleeding in the digestive tract, and various organ issues relating to these tissues losing blood.

Paget's Disease (pag-its)

A cellular disease. Bones will become deformed and will break down quickly. The old bone that breaks down will be replaced by new bones that are not properly organized. Fractures are likely to develop. Arthritis may also develop in some parts of the body. Some bones may also become thick. Paget's disease is likely to develop in the bone, although it may also develop in the breast and genital areas where some conditions may become rough or hard.

Pancoast Tumor

A bronchogenic tumor. The condition may negatively influence the sulcus region.

Parinaud's Syndrome (pair-in-oddz)

Enlargement of the lymph node. The condition develops on the same side that conjunctivitis may develop.

Parkinson's Disease

A degenerative central nervous system disorder. The condition impacts the motor system and will cause difficulties in how the CNS produces cells. This may lead to shaking and slow movements alongside difficulties walking. Some thinking or behavioral problems may also develop. Dementia can occur in some cases, although this occurs more in the later stages of the condition. This is believed to be a genetic condition, although those who are exposed to some pesticides and those who have experienced intense head injuries may be at high risk.

Peutz-Jegher's Syndrome (poot-z- jey-gurz)

When melanin pigments develop on the lips, mouth, hand, and genitals. This may also include polyps that develop in the small intestine.

Peyronie's Disease (pey-ron-eez)

When the connective tissue in the penile area is disrupted. Scar tissue will form in a sheath of tissue that surrounds the corpora cavernosa. The condition triggers pain and an unusual curve in the penile. Shortening may also develop in the organ. The condition becomes more likely to occur with age.

Pick's Disease

When the frontotemporal lobe degenerates. The proteins develop in the neurons, thus producing Pick bodies that stain the brain tissue. The condition may cause degeneration of the tissue. This is a form of dementia that progresses over time and is similar to Alzheimer's.

Plummer-Vinson Syndrome

Sideropenic dysphagia. A person experiences difficulty swallowing. Anemia relating to an iron deficiency may also develop. Iron supplements may help treat the condition, although a surgical procedure to widen the esophagus may be recommended for better results.

Pompe's Disease (pomp-eez)

A metabolic disorder. Also called glycogen storage disease type II. Muscle and nerve cells are damaged due to glycogen and lysosome developing in the body. The lysosomal acid alpha-glucosidase enzyme will not function properly. This may trigger myopathy, a condition where the muscles progressively become weaker. The nervous system and the heart may be negatively influenced by the condition.

Pott's Disease

A form of tuberculosis. The condition develops outside the lungs. The issue may be noticed in the vertebrae. The thoracic and lumbar vertebrae will develop issues where the bone structure deteriorates. The condition may be noticed through an elevated erythrocyte sedimentation rate.

Potter's Complex

Also referred to as the Potter sequence. The baby may not have enough exposure to amniotic fluid while in the uterus. The condition may produce clubbed feet, pulmonary hypoplasia, and cranial issues. Renal diseases may also trigger the issue.

Ramsay Hunt Syndrome

A condition that is a zoster infection in the facial nerve. This will produce palsy in the tissue. Type 1 syndrome is a progressive ataxia and tremors developing. Type 2 involves facial paralysis and ear pain alongside vesicles forming on the face and in the ear area. Type 3 syndrome involves the deep palmar branch in the ulnar nerve being directly influenced to where the tissue will weaken.

Raynaud's Syndrome (rey-nodz)

An arterial condition. Spasms will develop in the arteries reducing blood flow. The condition will impact the extremities, although the nose and ears may be involved. The condition causes the impacted area to become white and blue with numbness and pain developing. The area will then become red as blood flow returns to the area. The condition is triggered by cold conditions or stresses. An episode may last for a few hours in some instances.

Reiter's Syndrome (rye-turz)

Reactive arthritis. Inflammatory arthritis. This develops as the condition patient experiences inflammation due to an infection in another part of the body. Bacteria will travel along the body and can produce an infection in the impacted area. It is difficult to consider the original cause. (Note: The condition is usually referred to as "reactive arthritis" as a means of disavowing Hans Conrad Julius Reiter's involvement with the condition; Reiter was a member of the German Nazi party who conducted experiments in concentration camps. Some doctors may still use the name 'Reiter's syndrome' when discussing the condition because of simplicity or familiarity.)

Rett's Syndrome (rets)

A brain disorder. The MECP2 on the X chromosome mutates triggering seizures and scoliosis. A patient may experience a small head size and delayed growth. The condition develops in girls. Boys may experience a similar mutation, but they will die not long after birth. A genetic test may be required to confirm the condition.

Reye's Syndrome (rayz)

Encephalopathy. A person may experience changes in how the liver functions with the issue impacting the brain. The condition may develop following a viral infection. A person may experience seizures and significant personality changes as well as a possible loss of consciousness.

Riedel's Thyroiditis (rye-dellz)

Chronic thyroiditis. This may be due to the IgG4 compound producing excess plasma cells.

Rotor Syndrome

A benign bilirubin condition. The liver appears normal, but the gallbladder may be easier to notice due to jaundice developing in the area.

Saint's Triad

The development of diverticular disease in the colon, a hiatal hernia, and gallstones.

Schilder's Disease (sch-il-durz)

The neurodegenerative disease develops mainly in children, although it can occur in adults. This is a form of multiple sclerosis that can trigger dementia, balance issues, and poor attention.

Shaver's Disease

Lung fibrosis. The lungs are impaired due to excess aluminum inhalation.

Sheehan's Syndrome (she-hanz)

Postpartum pituitary necrosis. The condition develops due to blood loss and hypovolemic shock that occurs during and after the childbirth process. It may also be called Simmond's Syndrome.

Sipple's Syndrome (sip-pullz)

Multiple endocrine neoplasia type 2. A condition where tumors develop in the endocrine system. The tumors are not always malignant, but they can occur in various glands like the adrenal, parathyroid, and thyroid glands. This may trigger deformities in the tumors and may keep the tissues from being able to function normally.

Sjogren Syndrome (sig-roe-grin)

An autoimmune disorder. The moisture-generating glands are directly influenced. The glands will become weak and unable to produce the necessary moisture. The disorder will cause a dry mouth and dry eyes. A person may also be at a higher risk of developing lymphoma due to the condition.

Stargardt Disease (star-gart)

A retinal disease. The ABCA4 gene is directly influenced so that the retina will become weak with age. The condition develops in childhood in many cases. The eye will experience an elevated loss of vision.

Still's Disease

A form of juvenile arthritis. The body does not have an appropriate rheumatoid factor.

Sutton's Disease

An ulcerative condition. Benign ulcers or aphthae are frequently formed in the mouth. The patient is otherwise healthy. This may also be referred to as canker sores, although, the issue is developed due to a T cell-originated immune response that is influenced by the body's functionality.

Takayasu's Arteritis (tok-ah-yah-sooz)

Vasculitis. The aorta and pulmonary arteries are influenced by the vascular tissues becoming overly narrow. The body will not produce enough radial or ulnar pulses. The condition occurs mainly among those of Asian descent. Women are at an elevated risk.

Tay-Sachs Disease (tay-saks)

A genetic disorder. The body's nerve cells in the brain and spinal cord will slowly be destroyed. The condition will develop around three to six months after birth. The baby is unable to run, sit, or crawl. Seizures and hearing loss will also develop in some cases. This may be a deadly condition, although any cases where the disease develops later in life will be milder in intensity. The HEXA gene on chromosome 15 should be tested to identify a possible mutation, as the condition may be passed on through one's parents.

Tourette's Syndrome (tour-etz)

A neurodevelopmental condition. A person will develop various verbal and motor tics that will consistently happen. This may include sudden tics that will develop in one's muscles. Such tics may appear many times in a day. The cause of the condition is unknown, and there are no tests available to identify the condition in a patient.

Turner Syndrome

When a woman is missing part of an X chromosome. This may result in a woman developing a short statue, swelling in the hands, and a webbed neck. Hormonal treatment is required to support the development of breasts and menstrual periods. This may be referred to in some reports at 45,X or 45,X0 to specify the fact that the woman has 45 chromosomes versus the 46 that most people have.

Valentino's Syndrome (val-in-teen-ohs)

Pain that develops in the right lower part of the abdomen. A duodenal ulcer may develop with the ulcer perforating. The condition may cause an infection if not treated properly. Intense abdominal pain may develop when the condition develops.

Vincent's Infection

May also be called tonsillitis. The tonsils will become more visible and inflamed.

Von Gierke Disease (gear-kuh)

Glycogen storage diseases type I or GSD I. The body cannot store glycogen properly. The enzyme glucose-6-phosphatase does not function properly in this condition.

Von Hippel-Lindau Disease (von-hip-pull-lin-dow)

Familial cerebello retinal angiomatosis. A genetic condition. Benign tumors and some cysts may develop in the brain. The retina is likely to detach.

Von Willebrand's Disease (will-brand)

A blood-clotting condition. The body is unable to produce the von Willebrand factor or protein needed for supporting how platelets can secure themselves to one another. A person who has vWF totals of 30 to 50 IU/dL may be diagnosed as having the condition.

Warthin's Tumor (war-thins)

A cystic tumor in the salivary gland. The benign tumor is often found in those who frequently smoke cigarettes. The parotid gland may be influenced.

Watson Syndrome

When small nodules are produced on the iris. Noticeable veins and discoloration may develop. The disorder may influence the structure of the eye and may result in vision loss in the most significant cases.

Weil's Disease (whiles)

An infection of the Leptospira bacteria. Headaches may develop, although the most significant concern is a pulmonary hemorrhage forming.

Whipple's Disease (whip-pulls)

A disease caused by the Tropheryma whipplei bacterium. The body is unable to absorb its nutrients properly. The condition may influence the entire body, but some specific regions like the heart and brain may be impacted more than others. Weight loss and diarrhea may develop in most cases, although not all people will experience these problems.

Williams Syndrome

A genetic condition. The issue may trigger a large forehead and full cheeks alongside a short nose. A person could also experience a slight intellectual disability and may struggle with some visual-spatial functions. Others may develop hypercalcemia and heart-related conditions. The condition occurs when 27 genes from one of the chromosome 7s are deleted.

Werner Syndrome (wur-nur)

Adult progeria. A person experiencing premature aging. A person will grow and develop appropriately during childhood but will eventually develop Werner syndrome after puberty. The regular growth spurt associated with adolescence may not be noticed. A person may develop a reduced lifespan with the most common cause of death being a cardiovascular disease issue or some form of cancer. This is a genetic condition.

Medical Signs

Eponymous medical signs may be reported in some diagnostic reviews of patients. A medical sign refers to a sign of something that has developed. The conditions may be named for the doctors who first identified and described these, although they may also be named for a famous person who expressed one of these signs in the past.

Aaron Sign

Pain in the epigastrium when a person applies regular pressure. This is a sign of appendicitis.

Addis Count (add-iss)

A measurement of the number of cells in urine. This is based on a measure of urine produced within 24 hours.

Apgar Score (ap-gar)

A test on a newborn to identify how healthy the newborn is upon birth.

Aschheim-Zondek Test (ash-heye-m zon-dik)

A review of how well the female body's urine may respond. The test may identify compounds that can confirm that she is pregnant and that her pregnancy is running forward accordingly without complications.

Auer rod (our)

A cytoplasmic change in a myeloblast. The sign suggests that a person has acute myeloid leukemia.

Auspitz's Sign (os-pitz)

Bleeding that develops when scales are removed from a wart or a spot suspected to be associated with psoriasis.

Bainbridge Reflex (bain-bridge)

An increase in heart rate when the blood volume increases.

Bancroft's Sign (ban-krofts)

Pain on the anterior part of the calf during compression. The lateral area of the tissue will not experience any pain in this case. The condition can identify if deep vein thrombosis has developed.

Barlow's maneuver (bar-lowz)

When the hip experiences adduction. This may be a sign of hip dysplasia or dislocation.

Bart Hemoglobin

When the alpha-globin genes are not found in the blood. This is used when testing a stillborn child to identify the possible cause of death.

Bastian-Bruns Sign (bas-tee-in brunz)

The loss of muscle tone under a lesion. The condition may be a sign of spinal cord transection.

Beau's Lines (boze)

Transverse ridges that appear on the nails. The ridges can suggest that someone has experienced a form of trauma.

Beck's triad

Hypotension elevated central venous pressure, and heart sounds that feel removed. This includes the beats not coming too close to one another. This is a sign of cardiac tamponade.

Becker's sign

When the retinal arteries appear visible as they pulsate. This may suggest thyrotoxicosis.

Bezold-Jarisch reflex

Apena or bradycardia. These may develop due to a person using certain alkaloids.

Bitot's spots (by-tots)

Keratin appears visible in the conjunctiva. These include spots that are much darker than the white tissue associated with the conjunctiva. This may be a sign a person does not have enough vitamin A in the body.

Blumberg Sign (blum-burg)

When the body feels tender following a surgical procedure. The condition suggests the patient may develop peritonitis.

Braxton Hicks contraction (brax-tin hix)

False labor. Unusual contractions may develop in a woman's body during the middle part of the first trimester. This may suggest that the woman's pregnancy is developing normally and without any possible risks involved.

Broca aphasia (bro-cah)

Expressive aphasia. This may include concerns around parts of the brain where the organ is not functioning or developing accordingly.

Budin's sign (bue-din)

Brast milk that moves into a sterile pad and includes pus. This may be noted through some blood or yellow that come through the tissue. This may be a sign of mastitis.

Bruit de Roger (bru-eet)

A noticeable murmur in the heart. A ventricular septal defect may be noticed in this case.

Brushfield spots (brush-field)

Small gray or white spots around the iris. These may suggest that a person has developed Down syndrome.

Carvallo's sign (car-val-oh)

When the murmur in the heart becomes more intense following inspiration. The patient may be experiencing tricuspid regurgitation.

Celsus signs (sel-sus)

Signs that a person is experiencing inflammation. This may include redness, swelling, and pain in the area. Heat may also be felt in the impacted region.

Chaddock Reflex (chad-ock)

The big toe on the foot extending. A lesion may develop in the region.

Comby Sign (come-bee)

White patches formed on the gingiva. The child who shows this condition may be at risk of rubeola.

Coombs Test (coombs)

An analysis of how blood cells are formed. A fluorescent compound is applied to the blood sample to identify antibodies. The test identifies possible anemia-related issues, although it can also identify hemolytic anemia.

Curschmann spirals (kursh-min)

Spinal mucus plugs found in what a person expectorates. The condition is a sign that a person is experiencing difficulties due to asthma.

Dahl's Sign (dollz)

Calluses forming on the thighs. The calluses may develop from a person leaning the elbows on the thighs. The issue suggests a person may have COPD.

De Musset's Sign

When a person's head nods alongside the heartbeat. This may suggest that the person has an aortic condition where the aorta is no longer producing blood as well as it needs to.

Forchheimer spots (for-shy-mur)

A series of red spots on the soft palate. A patient may have rubella.

Frank's sign

An ear crease developing with a slight bend on the outside part. The bend may be a sign that a person has a high risk of developing heart disease.

Froment's sign

A patient holds a piece of paper between the thumb and index finger. If they are unable to grip it while someone tries to remove it, the patient may be at risk of developing ulnar nerve palsy.

Goodell's Sign (good-dells)

When the vaginal region of the cervix starts to soften. This occurs during the first trimester of pregnancy and suggests a woman is having a healthy pregnancy at the beginning.

Harrison's groove (hair-eh-sins)

A rib deformity developing around the lower part of the rib cage. The patient may develop rickets. Also called Harrison's sulcus.

Hutchinson's freckle (hut-chin-sins)

A considerable amount of facial pigmentation. This may suggest that a person is likely to develop melanoma. The pigmentation produced is a precancerous condition.

Hutchinson's pupil

Dilation in the pupil on the side of a lesion. The nerve in the area may develop excess compression. The concern suggests that the oculomotor nerve in the brain may not be functioning normally.

Hutchinson's sign

A lesion on the top of the nose. The condition is a sign of herpes zoster virus.

Hutchinson's teeth

When the incisors are spaced wide apart from one another. A few notched biting surfaces may appear. The incisors are also small in size. The patient may have developed syphilis. Nerve deafness and interstitial keratitis may also occur in this case.

Kehr's sign (carez)

Pains in the left shoulder without any prior fatigue developing in the tissue. The patient may be experiencing a ruptured spleen that has caused veins that head towards the left shoulder to become intense.

Ladin's sign (layd-inz)

A softened uterus. The tissue shows that the woman is experiencing a normal pregnancy. The sign may be identified at any time in the pregnancy to confirm the proper development of the unborn child.

Levine's sign (le-veenz)

When the patient clenches their fist over the chest while talking about the pain they are experiencing. The patient may be experiencing a myocardial infarction. The event occurs mainly as a natural reaction to feeling intense pain in the region.

Lombard effect

An effect where a person's voice rises in volume when they speak in a noisy environment. The effect may be noticed in cases where a person has hearing difficulties. This could also include a person's possible reactions to simulated deafness.

Markle's sign

Pains around the lower quadrant of the abdomen. The pain may develop when a person drops down after standing on one's toes or heels. The condition may be a sign of appendicitis.

Mayne's sign

The diastolic blood pressure drop of about 15 mmHg after the arm is raised. The patient may experience an aortic insufficiency.

Means-Lerman scratch

When a systolic heart murmur develops. This may be due to hyperthyroidism.

Mobius sign (moe-bee-us)

When the patient is unable to maintain the convergence of one's eyes. This could be a problem with the thyroid gland being too active or productive. That is, the patient has hyperthyroidism or thyrotoxicosis.

Muller's sign (moo-lurz)

When the uvula appears to be pulsating. The patient may have aortic difficulties.

Nikolsky's sign (nick-ole-skeez)

When the epidermis appears to break apart due to pressure. The condition may be a sign of a skin condition where tissues start to fatigue or break apart. This includes white tissues coming off the surface.

Palla's Sign (pal-ahs)

An enlarged right descending pulmonary artery. A chest x-ray is required to identify the condition. The patient may experience a pulmonary embolism due to the condition.

Patrick's test

The external rotation of the hip may be painful. The patient will develop inflammation in the sacroiliac joints or sacroiliitis.

Schilling test (shill-ing)

A test to identify vitamin B12 levels. The test may find that a person has pernicious anemia or a condition where the body is not absorbing nutrients properly.

Sister Mary Joseph nodule

A lymph node appears in the umbilicus. The node appears to be protruding or more noticeable than others. The condition indicates that a person has a concern in the abdominal region that is keeping the area from functioning properly.

Todd's paresis

When a person develops weakness for as long as 48 hours after the seizure takes place. The doctor may determine through this that the patient has a condition that includes intense fatigue and wear that can happen due to a seizure.

Surgical Procedures

Eponymous surgical procedures are named for the people who initially performed them or the patient that first went through the procedure. These procedures require extremely specific steps and processes to ensure that the patient's body is handled properly.

Bankart repair (ban-kart)

An orthopedic process. Frequent cases of shoulder dislocation are resolved as the joint capsule is sutured to the glenoid labrum. The practice keeps the shoulder from potentially moving.

Collis gastroplasty (col-is gas-troe-plas-tee)

The esophagus is stretched to elongate the tissue, thus improving how the tissue may function.

Fontan procedure (fon-tan)

A process that treats heart-related conditions in children. This is specifically for univentricular hearts. The procedure will move venous blood from the inter and superior vena cava to the pulmonary arteries. The process keeps the right ventricle from being a concern.

Hadfield's procedure (had-feel-dz)

The surgical removal of ducts in the breast tissue, including ducts that may produce milk. The treatment is to manage duct ectasia.

Heller myotomy (hel-lur)

The lower esophageal sphincter is cut to allow food to move into the patient's stomach. The surgery is for patients who struggle with keeping their muscles relaxed when attempting to consume foods.

Kausch-Whipple procedure (kosh whip-pul)

A pancreaticoduodenectomy. Cancerous tumors found on the top part of the pancreas are removed. The process requires the duodenum, jejunum, and gallbladder to be removed. A small portion of the stomach may also be involved. The procedure assists in preserving as much of the pancreas as possible. The pancreas, stomach, and bowel will be secured together following the extensive procedure.

Paul's Operation

A procedure where the colon is reorganized outside the abdomen. The procedure is for correcting issues where the colon is not functioning properly.

Smith's operation

The removal of a cataract within the lens. The procedure is an intracapsular procedure into the eyeball prior to the cataract possibly developing.

Tommy John surgery

A procedure where the ulnar collateral ligament or the triangular band along the medial part of the elbow is restored. The tissue is restored to enhance the functionality of the elbow. The procedure is typically completed for those who have undergone extreme fatigue and wear in the tissue, particularly baseball pitchers.

Wertheim's operation (wurth-heye-mz)

A total hysterectomy to eliminate cervical cancer. The hysterectomy will ensure the cervix, both ovaries, and fallopian tubes are removed with the cancerous tissues.

Chapter 27 – Medications and Medical Compounds

Many of the terms that you will encounter will refer to the medications used in a medical facility. These include medications that are necessary for treating certain types of functions and activities in the body. This chapter concentrates on some of the more common medications that may be prescribed by physicians. Notice some of the suffixes that relate to medications. These suffixes and prefixes refer to the ways certain compounds work.

Note: Some of the drugs listed in this chapter are ones that were originally designed to treat certain conditions, but they have been repurposed in recent time to help with other conditions. These include drugs to treat high blood pressure being used to treat erectile dysfunction. Consult a copy of the Physicians' Desk Reference for more information on how these medications work and how they are provided to patients.

Suffixes

The follow suffixes involve the ways drugs may be offered to the body. The suffixes are most important to identify the name of the drug. While the root word may indicate the part of the body that the medication will treat, sometimes the root or prefix will indicate the chemical materials.

These suffixes may be the generic names of some of these drugs. Some medications may be known better for their brand names. Many of these brand names will be listed later in this chapter.

Suffix	Type of Drug and Its Functionality
afil	Phosphodiesterase inhibitor or PDE. The drug inhibits the production of the PDE enzyme. This improves upon pulmonary vasodilation, although it may also influence how penile muscles can relax when treating erectile dysfunction.
asone	Corticosteriod. The drug is produced in the adrenal cortex. This is needed to support metabolic activities and can treat inflammation in the body.
bicin	Antineoplastic. The drug prevents the development of a neoplasm. This may also inhibit the processes where neoplasms are produced. This can be used when a tumor has to be treated.
bital	A barbiturate. The drug is based on a barbituric acid. This is a sedative that assists people to fall asleep. The drug may be dangerous if taken for too long, as a barbiturate will work stronger than many other over-the-counter tablets.

caine	Anesthetic. The local anesthetic is applied on a part of the body to control the development of pains in the body.
cillin	Penicillin. This is an antibiotic that is used to treat conditions relating to the staph and strep bacteria forms.
cycline	Tetracycline and other related compounds. The drug will treat acne and various skin infections.
dazole	An anthelmintic. The drug treats parasites and will kill parasitic worms or other things that have infested the body. The drug kills the parasite and stuns and kills it. The drug should not cause much damage to the host of the parasite. Some drugs with the –dazole suffix may also work as antibiotic and antibacterial drugs.
dipine	Calcium channel blocker. The compound will prevent calcium from moving through calcium channels in the body. The medication focuses on reducing blood pressure levels.
dronate	Bone resorption inhibitor. This is a bisphosphonate, a drug that will prevent bones from becoming weak. Patients with osteoporosis may benefit from the use of this drug option.
eprazole	Proton pump inhibitor or PPI. The drug reduces the amount of stomach acid production in the body. This may control how the acid is generated and works best in cases where a patient experiences a substantial amount of acid in the body. The drug use should be monitored and stopped if any symptoms are noticed that happen because of not having enough acid in the body.
fenac	Non-steroidal anti-inflammatory drug or NSAID. The drug prevents blood clots and pains in the body. This may also reduce inflammation if enough is taken or the drug is used for a while. The drug may trigger an elevated risk of GI bleeding and ulcers. Some patients may also develop kidney-related issues if the medication is used for too long.
floxacin	Quinolone. This is an antibiotic that treats bacterial infections. This may be provided in veterinary hospitals to treat bacterial infections in animals and to help facilitate animal husbandry efforts. However, the amount of the medication to be provided should be determined based on the size of the patient and how well that entity can handle the drug.
gliptin	Antidiabetic. The DPP-4 enzyme is controlled in the process. The drug's goal is to produce healthy control.

glitazone	Thiazolidinedione. The drug lowers the body's ability to resist insulin, thus controlling how well blood sugar levels may be managed by the body. The drug helps those who have Type II diabetes. New fat cells may be supported by the medication, thus lowering the body's blood glucose levels while the body has an easier time with managing glucose and insulin stores.
iramine	Antihistamine. The drug will treat allergy symptoms like a runny nose, sneezing, watery eyes, and other forms of irritation. The drug prevents the production of histamines that trigger allergic reactions from exposure to certain allergens.
lamide	Carbon anhydrase inhibitor. The drug stops the production of hydrogen and bicarbonate atoms in the body. Therefore, the risk of carbon dioxide and water impacting the renal tube will be controlled. The renal system can remove water, potassium, sodium, and other compounds safely without worry.
mab	Monoclonal antibody. The antibody is produced by immune cells that have been cloned from a parent cell. These will bind to the same bacterial compound that has to be neutralized. The medication is mainly for cancer treatments as the new antibodies produced imitate the immune system's ability to attack cancer cells. In particular, the antibody will secure itself on an antigen that may be more prominent than what is found on a cancer cell.
mustine	Antineoplastic agent. The compound will stop the development of a tumor or neoplasm. This may control various cancer forms, including some cancers that may have spread to other parts of the body.
mycin	An antibacterial agent.
nacin	Anticholinergic. The compound blocks the movement of acetylcholine, a neurotransmitter, from passing through the central and peripheral nervous systems. The agents will block nerve impulses and will prevent the transmitter from getting to the proper nerve cells where receptors may be found.
nazole	Antifungal. The drug will control any fungal infections that have developed in the body. The drug is typically administered orally, although some antifungals may be administered through a topical application.

olol	Beta-blocker. The compound treats hypertension and may protect a heart from having a second heart attack after it has experienced one earlier. This may also control unusual heart rhythms.
olone	Corticosteroid or anabolic steroid depending on the drug.
onide	Corticosteroid.
oprazole	PPI.
parin	Anticoagulant. This is a blood thinner that reduces the likelihood of the blood to clot as much as usual.
phylline	Bronchodilator. The drug will dilate the bronchi and bronchioles, thus reducing the possible resistance that may develop in the body's airways. Airflow will move into the lungs. The medication may come in a traditional oral form, but some appliances that assist in sudden breathing issues may also work provided the proper medicine is added in the compound.
pramine	Tricyclic antidepressant or TCA. The drug controls symptoms of depression, although the drug works best when consumed at bedtime. The drug may trigger weight gain.
pred	Corticosteroid.
pril	Angiotensin-converting-enzyme or ACE inhibitor. The drug treats hypertension and congestive heart failure. As the ACE enzyme is stopped, blood vessels can dilate to keep blood pressure down.
profen	An NSAID.
ridone	Antipsychotic. This may be a major tranquilizer that controls psychotic episodes, including problems relating to paranoia or hallucinations.
sartan	Angiotensin II receptor antagonist or ARB. This is a receptor blocker that controls hypertension and may help manage heart failure-related conditions.
semide	Loop diuretic. The diuretic will enter the kidney and assist in the production and release of water. The drug is necessary in cases where the body is unable to manage some treatments.
setron	Serotonin 5-HT3 receptor antagonist. The drug controls the vagus nerve and other parts of the brain by managing the ways serotonin may be produced. Some of these drugs may also operate as antinauseants.

statin	Statin. The drug will reduce cholesterol levels in the blood. The drug may also be called an HMG-CoA reductase inhibitor.
tadine	Antihistamine. Some drugs in this form may also be used as antivirals and may be a part of drugs that can control flu-like symptoms.
terol	Bronchodilator.
thiazide	Thiazide diuretic. This may also be called a water pill.
tinib	Antineoplastic. This is a kinase inhibitor that prevents the development of neoplasms and may control ones that have already grown.
trel	Progestin. The drug is a female hormone solution.
tretin	Retinoid or dermatologic agent.
triptan	Antimigraine. The drug is for those who regularly experience intense headaches, particularly migraine headaches.
tyline	Tricyclic antidepressant or TCA.
vir	Antiviral. This may include a drug that treats specific viral infections like herpes, hepatitis, HIV, CMV, or the flu.
vudine	Antiviral.
zepam	Benzodiazepine. This is a psychoactive drug that reduces anxiety and may be used as a sedative or anticonvulsant.
zodone	Antidepressant.
zolam	Benzodiazepine.
zosin	Alpha-blocker.

Prefixes

Although there are not many, there are a few prefixes that may be identified when reviewing medications. These include medications that will have specific functions.

Prefix	Type of Drug and Its Functionality
cef, ceph	Cephalosporin. The antibiotic drug will inhibit the development of bacteria by attacking the enzymes in their cellular walls. The process ensures bacterial cells will not be likely to divide.
cort	Corticosteroid.

parin	Antithrombotic. The drug prevents blood clots from developing. This may be used when treating a blood clot or an acute thrombus, but this is best for preventing future clots from developing.
pred	Corticosteroid. This type of drug may assist in supporting muscles and can keep the muscles from wearing out during a significant medical episode.
sulfa	Antibiotic. This may also be an anti-inflammatory drug that will control the risk of infections.
tretin	A form of vitamin A.
vir	Antiviral. The type of virus the drug treats varies by the product.

Brand Name Drugs

A report on medications in your treatment space may refer to specific brand names. Some professionals will refer to medications by their brand names because they are easier to write and may be more prominently known.

Brand names may be used to refer to other drugs that have become available on the generic market. Generic drugs may be referred to as "Generic For (name of brand name drug)." Generics are popular for being cheaper and for including the same active ingredients as the brand names. Generics are only available after a certain time period has passed and the copyright protection for the manufacturer for the original brand name drug has expired.

The following list is a sample of the brand name drugs that you might encounter. This list is based on the more popular drugs.

Note: Depending on the doctor's recommendation or the patient's preference, there might be times when a person will require the brand name of a drug instead of the generic equivalent. This may be due to some concerns about the quality of generic drugs and if they include the same ingredients.

Brand Name	**Purpose of Drug**
Altace (Ramipril)	An ACE inhibitor for the treatment of high blood pressure and congestive heart failure.
Amaryl (glimepiride)	An anti-diabetic medication for the treatment of Type II diabetes.
Ambien (zolpidem)	For the treatment of insomnia. May also be available in the Edular, Zolpimist, and Intermezzo brands. The product may include a controlled release option.

Ativan (lorazepam)	For the treatment of seizures and conditions that trigger them, including epilepsy. This may also be prescribed before a surgical procedure to control anxiety. Also available as Lorazepam Intensol.
Calan SR (verapamil SR)	A standard release drug. The product is a calcium channel blocker and antihypertensive drug. This may be used as a treatment for arrhythmia and angina.
Cardizem (diltiazem)	A calcium channel blocker for angina. Also available as Tiazac and Taztia. This may be found in an extended-release form.
Celexa (Citalopram)	A selective serotonin reuptake inhibitor or SSRI. The drug will treat depression.
Coumadin (warfarin)	A blood thinner for preventing and treating blood clots. Also available as Jantoven.
Diabeta (glyburide)	An anti-diabetic medication for Type II diabetes. This is also available as Glynase.
Dilantin (phenytoin)	An anticonvulsant for the treatment of seizures. Found in an extended-release form. Some low-dosage options are available for children. Also available as Phenytek.
Effexor (venlafaxine)	For the treatment of nerve pain. This may also be prescribed for some anxiety disorders and for depression. An extended-release version is available.
Flonase (fluticasone)	A medication that is used through the nasal cavity. The compound is prepared and then sprayed into the cavity for proper treatment. This may also prevent asthma attacks from developing. The drug is a glucocorticoid. A low-dose version is available for children.
Fosamax (alendronic acid)	A bisphosphonate derivative. The drug may be injected once a month, although some oral options are also available. The drug treats and controls the development of osteoporosis. Paget's disease that impacts the bone may also be controlled. A Fosamax

Plus D variant that includes added vitamin D stores may also be offered to the patient.

Glucophage (metformin)

An anti-diabetic medication for the treatment of Type II diabetes. An extended-release option is available.

Glucotrol (glipizide)

Anti-diabetic medication for Type II diabetes. This cannot be consumed with alcohol. The drug enhances the pancreas' ability to produce insulin.

Hytrin (terazosin)

A urinary retention drug. The alpha-1 blocker will treat high blood pressure and BPH or an enlarged prostate.

Imitrex (sumatriptan)

A triptan medication. This may be used for controlling migraine and cluster headaches.

Lasix (furosemide)

A diuretic. This may treat fluid retention or edema that is caused by various organ diseases. The drug is known mainly for being something used by veterinarians to treat horses in horse racing activities, although smaller doses are safe for humans.

Lopid (gemfibrozil)

A cholesterol medication that will reduce blood triglyceride levels.

Mevacor (lovastatin)

A statin. Also available as Altoprev.

Micronase (glyburide)

Anti-diabetic medication for controlling Type II diabetes.

Norvasc (amlodipine)

Calcium channel blocker for the treatment of angina and hypertension.

Paxil (paroxetine)

Selectric serotonin reuptake inhibitor or SSRI that helps the treatment of depression, anxiety, and obsessive-compulsive disorder. This may also help women who are experiencing significant hormonal changes due to premenstrual conditions. This may be available in a controlled release form. Other brands include Pexeva and Brisdelle.

Pepcid (famotidine)

Antacid and antihistamine that targets ulcers and gastroesophageal reflux disease. The medication is available over the counter, although a high-dose version may also be offered through a prescription.

Pravachol (pravastatin)	A statin.
Prilosec (omeprazole)	Proton-pump inhibitor for heartburn and esophageal damages. This is available in small doses over the counter, but the most effective forms are only available through a prescription.
Prinivil (Lisinopril)	ACE inhibitor. The drug can reduce the risk of death if taken after a heart attack. Also available as Zestril.
Procardia (nifedipine)	A calcium channel blocker. This may reduce hypertension and angina. Available in an XL format.
Proventil (albuterol)	Bronchodilator. The medication is inhaled as necessary.
Prozac (fluoxetine)	SSRI for the treatment of depression and panic disorder. A weekly version of Prozac that releases slower is also available.
Retin-A (tretinoin)	A vitamin A-based material. This is available in an oral form for the treatment of some forms of leukemia. A topical solution is also available for the treatment of acne and other skin imperfections. This may also be found as Tretin-X.
Risperdal (risperidone)	An antipsychotic drug. The drug is for the treatment of schizophrenia and bipolar disorder. This may also be prescribed for those who have autism and experience constant fits of irritation.
Sonata (zaleplon)	A sedative. The drug is for those who regularly experience insomnia. The drug is a nonbenzodiazepine compound that can cause some significant interactions when consumed with alcohol.
Synthroid (levothyroxine)	A hormone medication that helps treat hypothyroidism, thyroid cancer, and enlarged thyroid gland-related issues. The drug is also needed when a patient has had one's thyroid gland removed for any reason.

Timoptic (timolol)	Beta-blocker. The drug helps treat high blood pressure and migraine headaches. This can also keep a person who has experienced a heart attack from being likely to have another. A liquid form for eye use is also available; the drug treats glaucoma in this form.
Toprol (metoprolol)	A beta-blocker that will treat high blood pressure and angina. The drug may be prescribed after a heart attack to reduce one's risk of dying from the event. The drug is available in an XL form and can also be found under the Lopressor name.
Tylenol-Codeine (acetaminophen)	A specialized version of the Tylenol acetaminophen drug that includes codeine. The drug is also known as Tylenol #3. The drug is for relieving intense pains from a surgical procedure or an extraction. The drug is an opioid and may be addictive if used for too long. This can cause respiratory illness if used for some time.
Ultram (tramadol)	A narcotic. This may help treat some pains. The drug can be extremely dangerous if used for too long as the drug can become addictive. This may also be deadly if used in high doses or if combined with alcohol.
Vasotec (enalapril)	A drug that treats kidney disease in diabetics and hypertension. The drug may be taken orally, although an intravenous solution may be used provided it is injected properly.
Ventolin (albuterol)	Bronchodilator. The drug may be inhaled as a beta-2-agonist.
Wellbutrin (bupropion)	A drug that helps people quit smoking. The drug may also treat depression that has been caused by seasonal affective disorder. Standard release and XL versions of the drug are available. Also offered as Zyban.
Xanax (alprazolam)	A sedative for the treatment of panic disorder. The drug must not be combined with other substances like alcohol or else the drug may trigger slow breathing rates and potentially become deadly.

Yasmin (drospirenone)	A birth control pill that has to be taken every day. The pill includes estrogen and progestin, two hormones that help to prevent pregnancies from developing. The pill can be found in many other brands like Aviane, Mircette, Levora, Levlite, Lessina, Aranella, and Nordette.
Zantac (ranitidine)	Antacid and antihistamine. The drug will prevent and treat heartburn and GERD among other issues that may be triggered by excess stomach acid. The drug also reduces the production of stomach acid. The drug can be found over the counter with some options with larger concentrations of ingredients available through a prescription.
Zestril (Lisinopril)	ACE inhibitor. This may treat hypertension and can reduce the risk of heart failure in a patient. Also available in Qbrelis.
Zocor (simvastatin)	A statin that treats cholesterol and triglyceride levels in the body.
Zoloft (sertraline)	A selective serotonin reuptake inhibitor. The drug will treat depression and obsessive-compulsive disorder among other mental concerns. This may particularly be prescribed for the treatment of social anxiety disorder.
Zovirax (acyclovir)	Antiviral drug. The drug controls herpes virus infections and can control genital herpes. The drug may also reduce the intensity of the chickenpox virus. Herpes sores and blisters may also be prevented, although the drug should not be interpreted as a cure for herpes.

Additional Terms For Medications

The following terms may be noticed when reviewing medications based on their names and how they are labeled. These terms may help you identify how to administer these medications or how these drugs will function. The terms may be listed on the medication packages and labels themselves, although some study of individual medications may be required to confirm that these compounds can work in the ways that they are promoted.

Capsule

A rectangular-shaped capsule that includes dry and powdered ingredients that are secured to enhance the ability of the body to absorb the capsule. A gelling agent, particularly protein, may be used to create the outside capsule.

CR

Controlled release. The drug takes a long time for its content to be administered.

Enteric-Coated

A tablet that is coated with a polymer. The polymer protects the contents of the drug to ensure the drug will not be harmed by the stomach acids. The drug will release accordingly and is effective even if stomach acids are present.

Injection

The drug has to be injected into the bloodstream. A hypodermic needle is required with a syringe. The compound should be pierced through the skin in an appropriate location involved with blood veins. A needle must be sterile to prevent a risk of infection.

IR

Immediate release. The entire dosage of the drug is released all at once after it is administered.

Intensol

A concentrated oral solution. The solution must be mixed with another liquid. This may be mixed with water or juice, although some semi-solid foods like a pudding or applesauce may be used. A dropper should be included with an intensol-based drug.

Intradermal

To be injected in between the epidermis and hypodermis. The medication is to be absorbed through the skin.

Intramuscular

The drug will be administered directly into a muscle. The administration is done with about 2 to 5 mL of medication at a time. The administration offers a faster absorption rate than what may be provided through subcutaneous injection or an intradermal injection.

Intranasal

An intranasal administration process is a medication applied locally in the nasal cavities and may also work systemically. This works best for the treatment of concerns relating to nasal congestion or allergy-related issues.

Infusion

Infusion is a process where a drug is transferred to the patient's circulatory system. This may be done intravenously by an arterial or subcutaneous administration process to improve the effectiveness of the drug.

Inhalation

An inhalation process is used when a person needs to take in medication but requires extra help due to the acids in the body. The inhalation process allows for the proper vapors involved with the drug to be controlled and added into the airways to treat various concerns. Most inhalation-based drugs will focus on airways.

Intravenous

This process for administering medication is also known as intravenous treatment. The process delivers a liquid compound to the body through a vein. This may be used in cases where the body requires immediate access to a medication and cannot handle the acids that may cause some medications to disintegrate. Due to the sensitive nature of a vein, the intravenous process requires a doctor to target the specific vein where the drug is to be administered.

Lotion

A lotion is designed for topical use. The lotion would include an active ingredient that is secured within a base that can be directly administered on an area. This is used for concerns relating to the skin. The lotion would have to be used carefully, as some lotions may produce adverse effects if they are applied on tissues where the lotion is not necessary.

Lozenge

A lozenge is a compound that comes in a diamond shape. The oral tablet is used mainly for sore throat-related issues. This may include some flavoring agents to make the compound easier for the person to consume.

Mouthwash

Mouthwash is a liquid that is applied in the mouth and then held passively. The liquid may also be swished around to cover more areas around the mouth. This is for dental or oral conditions. The mouthwash will likely have to be spewed out from the body after a bit of time. The patient should hold the mouthwash in the mouth for as long as prescribed.

MR

Modified release. Some parts of the drug may be administered prior to other parts. The timeframe for the compounds to be administered will vary based on the quality and compounds of the drug.

Nebulizer

The nebulizer is a material that will change medications from a liquid to a mist, thus making it easier for a person to inhale the drug into the lungs. The treatment is for cases where the airways are impacted and need some form of relief. A nebulizer may be used to treat various conditions relating to the lungs, although the compound will require enough of the medication for it to work effectively. Also, some nebulizers may be too large for people to transport.

ODT

Orally disintegrating tablet. The tablet will break down as it reaches the tongue. The tablet is not supposed to be swallowed, but rather applied on the tongue so it may dissolve. The tablet is for those experiencing dysphagia, a condition where a person is unable to swallow properly.

Ointment

Used topically. An ointment is different from a lotion in that the ointment is oily in texture. The ointment is to be rubbed on the skin to allow the targeted area to be treated. The same precautions should be taken for the process as what is taken for a lotion.

Oral

A drug that must be taken orally or by mouth. The patient must be able to swallow the drug without issues. A sip of water or another recommended fluid may be necessary to facilitate the swallowing process.

OROS

Osmotic-controlled release oral delivery system. A controlled release format where a hard tablet is utilized with a semi-permeable outside membrane included. A few small holes are produced by a laser. When the tablet moves through, water is absorbed into the medication through osmosis. The osmotic pressure will move the drug through the tablet openings. OROS is a trademark of the ALZA Corporation and may not be directly listed on all drugs that use this system.

Pastille

A candy drug. The pill is a drop, gummy, or other candy-like material that has the medicine liquefied and then solidified into a surface. The patient should chew the drug and allow it to dissolve in the mouth.

Sublingually

Under the tongue. The medication is applied under the tongue and allows it to dissolve there. The area under the tongue includes an extensive array of blood vessels that will absorb the medication. The process may help allow the body to take in more of the medication without the compound possibly breaking apart.

Suppository

A medication that enters through the anus and rectum. This medication is used when the colon or kidneys need to be treated. A doctor would have to administer the medication for the best results. The most common type of suppository is an enema, although that is used mainly to examine the bowels.

Suspension

A liquid that includes some of the drug inside, which has not been fully dissolved. The drug should be shaken or stirred before use to ensure the proper amount of drug is consumed every time it is used.

Syrup

A thick liquid that is a solution mixed in sugar in water. The syrup includes a large amount of dissolved sugars. The syrup may be supported with corn syrup to convert a compound into sugars that may be used in the body. It might take some time for the syrup to go through due to its thick texture.

XL

Extended-release. The body will take in the medication and the product will be released gradually. This may take some time for the medication to be fully used.

Side Effects

Different types of drugs have various side effects that may develop. These side effects can be complicated and hard to live with especially when planning medications for people and ensuring that they will get the most out of the medication.

Allergic Reaction

An allergic reaction occurs when a person consumes a drug and experiences something where the immune system attacks the body. The reaction may be a rash, itching, excess tear production, and sneezing. In some cases, the reaction might be hives and fever among other concerns. Some conditions may be significantly serious and could result in breathing difficulties. This includes situations where the person could be at risk of death.

The allergic reaction may develop due to a person having an allergy to a specific ingredient in the drug. The reaction may not always be due to the particular active ingredient included in the drug. This may be due to an interaction with a particular type of inactive ingredient that is included.

Bleeding Issues

Bleeding conditions may develop in some drugs. These include problems where a person may start bleeding internally. A person experiences leaks in the blood vessels or other tissues that struggle to maintain their blood stores. The problem might be a significant threat.

In other cases, it might be easy for a person to experience further bleeding due to the blood not being as likely to clot. The lack of clotting may be a threat to life.

Chemical Suppression

Some drugs may also suppress the production and usage of various chemicals in the body. These include many neurotransmitters or enzymes needed for regular functionality. For instance, dry mouth may develop from some medications because they have chemicals that stop the mouth being hydrated and does not support saliva production from developing properly or normally.

Drug Interactions

A drug may be influenced by another medication that is being taken. This includes cases where one drug might become exaggerated or minimal in function after a second drug is taken around the same time.

Alcohol Influence

Alcohol may cause some drugs to become more intense. Alcohol can trigger a drug to be active and potentially harm the body. This is especially the case when it comes to some drugs used for controlling diabetes. The multiplication effect involved with alcohol can cause some drugs to become deadly.

Excess Dosage

Excess dosage risks are critical. The dosage of medication should be measured carefully to ensure the drug is consumed properly. The added dosage could potentially be deadly. Liquid or nasal medications need to be measured precisely.

The Food and Drug Administration requires all drug manufacturers to provide full disclosure about the precautions involved with the drugs.

Chapter 28 – Body Features

While the individual physical systems in the human body are important to understand, individual features in the body may also develop. The following chapter focuses on basic body features to identify many ways the body operates. These terms may also be used in writing reports that identify the location of a physical condition.

Anatomical Planes

An anatomical plane refers to a certain section in the body according to a series of perpendicular and parallel lines. These lines go across the body. The entire body is divided into a series of sections.

Coronal (coe-roe-nil)

The frontal plane, the coronal plane is a vertical line that divides the anterior and posterior parts of the body.

Midsagittal (mid-saj-it-ul)

The midsagittal plane is the midline of the body. This is a vertical longitudinal line that divides the left and right sides of the body.

Sagittal (saj-it-ul)

A sagittal plane is a vertical plane from the anterior to posterior parts of the body. The body will be separated from the left and right parts.

Transverse (trans-vurs)

The plane, in this case, is parallel to the ground. The upper half of the body is divided from the lower half at the waist.

Body Position

These positions refer to how the person's body is positioned during an exam or procedure. The positioning will be chosen according to the analysis that has to be done. The body may also be placed at different positions based on the area that needs to be examined.

Anatomic (an-ah-tom-ick)

The anatomic position is the most basic type of position that the body can be in. This is a review of the body when it is upright. The arms are on the sides with the palms are positioned forward. The feet are next to each other with the toes pointing forward. The position is used to identify any unusual cases where the patient's posture may be impacted or if there are any unusual features protruding. The patient's ability to maintain the anatomic position for a while may also be measured to see if that person is strong or weak or if they have a balance-related issue.

Erect (ee-wrekt)

The body is erect when the person stands upright. The person should attempt to stay as upright and tall as possible.

Fowler (fow-lur)

The patient starts the position as supine (lying on the back with face upward). The head is raised by about 18 inches. The knees are also elevated. This may help identify how well the body can respond to breathing-related activities.

Genupectoral (gen-ue-pec-tor-ul)

The patient is on their knees while on an examination surface. The head and upper part of the body will then be lowered to the surface. The chest and knees will carry most of the patient's weight. The process is used mainly for rectal exams, although this can also identify how well the patient is capable of maintaining their weight in that position.

Lateral Recumbent (re-kum-bint)

The patient is lying on one side with one leg slightly bent at the knee.

Lithotomy (lith-ot-oe-mee)

The person lies in the recumbent position and then keeps the thighs apart while the legs are drawn towards the abdomen.

Prone (pr-own)

When a person is lying face down. The abdomen should be flat on the surface.

Sims (sim-z)

The sims position is a side position where the patient is on their left side. The right thigh is pulled up toward the chest. The right knee should also be close to the chest.

Recumbent (re-cum-bint)

When the person lies on their back with the chest facing up. This may also be called a supine position. This is the procedure that is typically used for surgical procedures, although the positioning may vary based on the condition that has to be examined or tested.

Trendelenburg (tren-del-en-berg)

When the patient lies on their back and the legs are elevated higher than the head.

Nine Regions of the Abdomen and Pelvis

The precise location of a physical concern that a patient may experience can be listed on a doctor's report. The analysis will include details that may be listed as "Region I," "Region IV," or another option. The region is listed based on the particular features of the body at the subjected area. A report can include these region-based terms to identify specific concerns surrounding a patient's body and how a procedure or effort may be planned.

The nine regions are listed as Roman numerals. For instance, II on this list would be referred to in a report as Region II. The regions are labeled from top to bottom:

I. The right hypochondriac region. The gallbladder and the right lobe of the liver are in this section. This is the upper right part of the abdomen.

II. The epigastric region. The middle part of the liver and much of the stomach is included. The area below the rib cage is also included.

III. Left hypochondriac. The large intestine and part of the stomach can be found in this section. This is the upper left part of the abdomen.

IV. Right lumbar. Parts of both the small and large intestine may be noticed in this area. The area is directly under the right hypochondriac region.

V. Umbilical region. This is the direct middle part of the abdomen. The small intestine and a part of the transverse colon are in this area.

VI. Left lumbar. The colon and small intestine are in this section.

VII. Right inguinal or iliac region. The cecum and a part of the small intestine are in this section. This is around the bottom-most part of the abdominal and pelvic area.

VIII. Hypogastric. The urinary bladder and the end part of the small intestine are both in this section .

IX. Left inguinal or iliac. The small intestine and colon are in the region, but again only a portion of the tissues are in this section.

Cavities

Many reports will include details on the specific cavity in the body treatment or condition may be noticed. A cavity is a segment in the body that includes many of the critical organs that the body requires for survival. Here are cavities in the body:

Abdominal (ab-dom-in-ul)

Located in the abdomen. The stomach, intestines, kidneys, liver, spleen, pancreas, and gallbladder are located in this part of the body. This is one of the largest cavities.

Cranial (cray-nee-ul)

The cranial cavity is associated with the head and keeps the organs in the posterior part of the body secured. Therefore, the cavity is a dorsal space. The brain is in the cranial cavity.

Pelvic (pel-vick)

The cavity is in the pelvis. This is a ventral cavity for securing organs and where the urinary bladder and the body's reproductive system are protected.

Spinal (spy-null)

The spinal cord and the nerves that originate from the area are found in the region. All major segments of the spinal column are involved and it also includes support for producing the sensations that the body has.

Thoracic (thor-ack-ik)

The chest or thorax cavity. This is a ventral cavity, which means that it is in the anterior part of the body. The body's critical organs are secured in this area. The lungs and heart are secured alongside the trachea and esophagus at the top part.

Quadrants

Quadrants refer to the four areas in the abdominal region where a condition may develop. These are divided based on the upper or lower and right or left segments. The quadrant may be identified in a report with the following letters:

1. R or L for right or left

2. U or L for upper or lower

3. Q for the quadrant

Therefore, the RLQ is the right lower quadrant, and the LLQ is the left lower quadrant.

Each of these quadrants is critical for how it includes various points in the body. The RLQ is where parts of the intestines are found alongside the right part of the ureter. The LLQ features the left ureter and added parts of the intestines. The upper quadrants focus on the liver and surrounding organs in the area.

Chapter 29 – Tips For Studying Terms

The information in this guide is extremely detailed and useful. This final chapter will help you find ways how to study the terms and how you can work towards enhancing your ability to remember them.

1. Make sure you take notes as necessary.

Take notes on whatever you feel may be important. This includes notes on what an instructor talks about and the lessons being taught. Include as much information as possible in your notes, but try to ensure the data is kept clean and sensible so you can follow the content without a problem.

2. Plan a schedule to study your terms.

You can use a schedule that covers different aspects of the medical terms. This includes studying terms used for certain segments of the body or prefixes or suffixes. You should devote enough time to your studies for each section. More time will need to be spent studying terms that you are new to you.

3. Complete tests and quizzes online.

One of the main reasons people want to learn medical terms is so they can not only understand the content but also pass certification exams. You can use online quizzes and tests to help you test your knowledge of the terms and meanings you have been studying. Various quizzes can help you identify many terms that may need more study.

4. Look for possible cues.

Break a term down into its parts. Understanding the individual segments of a word can help you review the spatial considerations for body parts or other functions. Visual cues help you recall information by recognizing the links between the root word, the suffix, and the prefix.

5. Check for unique study tools that you can find online. You can find many useful tools that may work for your studies. These include various flashcard programs.

It is very easy to use study tools to make it easier to learn new terms. There are too many programs relating to these tools for you to consider, but the options that you can find are worth considering.

6. Take breaks.

As important as it is for you to study these terms, it is also important for you to ensure you don't try to study when you are overtired. You need to take breaks every once in a while to ensure you won't feel burned out. You can plan for breaks that you require within your schedule for studying.

7. Be willing to ask for help if you need it.

You'll need to work with other people if you're going to make the most out of your studies. The problem with trying to learn terms on your own is that you might struggle with all the complicated details. If you work with another person, you can help each other.

Teamwork can help you identify areas in which you are weak or are struggling to learn. You can also find ways to fix the problems surrounding what you understand. You may even come up with some new ideas to increase your ability to remember.

Conclusion

Your effort in understanding and remembering medical terms are important to your success. You will have to identify how these medical terms are created and how you can use them to communicate with other people.

The medical environment is a high-pressure field. People who are in the medical field must work with precision and care. This is to ensure that everyone involved uses the same terms for conditions and treatment. However, some words in the field may be extremely complex or easy to confuse. Understanding the roots, prefixes and suffixes, abbreviations, acronyms, and other terms in the field is vital to your success.

You will find that it is not difficult to make the most out of your studies when you have the knowledge you require. Knowing how these medical terms are created, how you can produce them, pronounce them, or determine the meanings is important to your success.

The most important thing to do when reviewing these terms is to know how every syllable means something unique.

Good luck in your efforts in getting the most out of your medical studies. You will discover through the work you put in that it will not be hard to go further with your efforts when moving forward with the work you want to do. More importantly, you will find that your work in the medical field will make a significant difference when you are able to contribute to helping people who are suffering.

Index

Printed in Great Britain
by Amazon